Deanne Anders was re... friends were still readin... knew she'd hit the jackp... of Harlequin Presents in ... local library. Years later she discovered the fun of writing her own. Deanne lives in Florida, with her husband and their spoiled Pomeranian. During the day she works as a nursing supervisor. With her love of everything medical and romance, writing for Mills & Boon Medical is a dream come true.

Juliette Hyland began crafting heroes and heroines in high school. She lives in Ohio, USA, with her Prince Charming, who has patiently listened to many rants regarding characters failing to follow their outline. When not working on fun and flirty happily-ever-afters, Juliette can be found spending time with her beautiful daughters and giant dogs, or sewing uneven stitches with her sewing machine.

THE REBEL DOCTOR'S SECRET CHILD

DEANNE ANDERS

FAKE DATING THE VET

JULIETTE HYLAND

MILLS & BOON

First published in Great Britain 2024
by Mills & Boon, an imprint of HarperCollins*Publishers* Ltd,
1 London Bridge Street, London, SE1 9GF

www.harpercollins.co.uk

HarperCollins*Publishers* Macken House, 39/40 Mayor Street Upper, Dublin 1, D01 C9W8, Ireland

The Rebel Doctor's Secret Child © 2024 Denise Chavers

Fake Dating the Vet © 2024 Juliette Hyland

ISBN: 978-0-263-32175-3

10/24

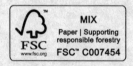

This book contains FSC™ certified paper and other controlled sources to ensure responsible forest management.

For more information visit www.harpercollins.co.uk/green.

Printed and Bound in the UK using 100% Renewable Electricity at CPI Group (UK) Ltd, Croydon, CR0 4YY

THE REBEL DOCTOR'S SECRET CHILD

DEANNE ANDERS

MILLS & BOON

This book is dedicated to all the medical staff
who volunteer their time at our local clinics, schools,
and with our local disaster teams.
Thank you for your service.

PROLOGUE

EXCITEMENT VIBRATED THROUGH Brianna Rogers as she followed the office manager, Sable, into the crowded conference room. With her arms loaded down with boxes of donuts, Brianna looked across the table at all the people she'd soon be working with. She'd done it. In just a few months, she'd be working as a certified nurse midwife. The opportunity for a residency at Nashville's Women's Legacy Clinic was one that she'd never imagined receiving. It was known as the premier women's clinic in the city, so the experience she'd receive here would be priceless.

As the door opened and a silver-haired man with kind blue eyes came in, the room went quiet. Bree rushed to her seat. She had only met the founder of the clinic, Dr. Jack Warner, once during an interview, but she admired the practice he'd built and especially the home for pregnant women in need of a safe place to stay that he had founded.

He took his seat at the end of the table then reached for the tablet Sable had told her contained the itinerary for the meeting.

"First off, I'd like to welcome two new colleagues. I

hope you've all met our new resident midwife, Brianna Rogers. She's a recent graduate of Vanderbilt and came to us highly recommended."

A man yelled, "Go Commodores," from across the room, taking the attention off her, something she appreciated. One of the midwives, Sky, waved at her from down the table. Bree waved back. Even with the unwanted attention, she was already feeling at home here.

"Also, I want you to welcome Dr. Knox Collins, who will be filling in for Dr. Hennison, who, I'm sure you all know, just welcomed another baby boy."

Bree's heart skipped a beat and her arms and face prickled with tiny pinpricks. No. It was impossible that he could be there. A roaring in her ears started as her eyes scanned the room, stopping when she saw a man with laughing gray eyes and a devilish smile that should have come with a warning.

Never in her wildest dreams would she have imagined herself stuck looking across the table at the man who had broken her sister's heart and left Bree to pick up the pieces. Especially since one of those pieces had been a newborn baby. She'd never forget the first time she'd heard that name. It had been when her phone rang. She hadn't spoken to her sister in months and was so happy to see her name on the display.

Suddenly, she was back there, eight years earlier. Brittany, her voice overflowing with a happiness Bree hadn't heart in years, laughing as she told Bree the news. "It's a girl, Bree. A beautiful baby girl. I have a daughter. You're an aunt."

Stunned, Bree didn't know what to say. Brittany had been pregnant? How was that possible without Bree knowing about it?

"Well, aren't you going to congratulate me?" her sister asked.

"Of course," Bree said, recovering from the shock of her sister's words. "Where are you?"

Bree listened closely as her sister explained how she'd gone into labor early and the baby was still in the hospital.

"Who's the father?" Bree asked, unable to hold back the question any longer. Brittany had been known to hook up with some less than desirable types in the past.

"It's Knox Collins, Gail and Charles Collins's son. But you can't tell anyone. Me. This baby. We mean nothing to him. He's messed up, Bree. He drinks and parties all the time. I don't want that for my daughter. Promise me you won't tell anyone, Bree. Promise me."

Bree had no choice but to agree. If Brittany thought the man would be a bad influence on her daughter, she had no choice but to believe her. She'd ask for more information the next time her sister called her.

But the next call she received wasn't from her sister. Instead, it was from the hospital. She could hear the woman's voice. "I'm sorry, Ms. Rogers, but there's been a terrible accident."

She told the woman that she was wrong. She'd just spoken with her sister only hours earlier. Her sister couldn't be gone.

She remembered holding her niece in her arms for the

first time, knowing it should have been Brittany standing there to take her baby home. Not Bree.

Overwhelming grief had threatened to overtake her then, but she pushed it back. Just like she had when she'd realized she was suddenly responsible for her sister's newborn baby. There was no time for grieving. Because if she let it take hold of her, she'd never climb out of the dark pit of it. She'd never be able to take care of the child who had no one else. Just like Bree had no one else but that child.

The noise of the room rose, bringing her back to reality as everyone around her stood up to leave.

Looking down the table she saw Knox accepting the greetings from the clinic's staff. How was it that he stood there, smiling and happy, going on with his life while her sister's life was cut so short?

Bree shook her head. No. She wouldn't let herself go there. Ally had to be her first priority. The little girl had given Bree a reason to keep on going for years now, to keep pushing to better herself so that she could provide a good life for her niece. And there was no way she was going to let some hotshot rebel doc like Knox Collins get in her way.

CHAPTER ONE

BRIANNA ROGERS WAS trying to ignore them. All of them. The giggling nurse with bouncy honey-blond curls Bree would give her already strained credit card to have, the anesthesia nurse whose toothpaste-ad smile could blind someone, and the drooling surgical tech whose no-nonsense attitude had turned disgustingly mushy. But most of all, she was trying to ignore the man in the middle of all three of them, Knox Collins.

From the moment Bree had attended her first staff meeting at Women's Legacy Clinic, she'd made it her priority to avoid Knox. For three months she had accomplished the impossible by managing to dodge the man whom she'd considered enemy number one for the past eight years. It looked like her luck had run out now, and the only thing she could do was pretend that he wasn't there.

Her teeth ground against each other when the blonde nurse giggled again at something Knox had said. She forced her eyes back to the computer screen in front of her and did her best to block out everyone else in the room.

Should she have turned down the opportunity that

Dr. Warner, Jack, had given her when she'd found out Nashville's own bad boy turned doctor was going to be there? Maybe, but how could she? With the amount of student loans she had and the cost of raising her niece, she was lucky to get the chance to do her midwife residency at the clinic. There was no way she could afford to turn down the opportunity. Not having to leave Nashville or change her niece's school had been a blessing and reduced the stress that always seemed to be right around the corner waiting to overwhelm her. Oh, she'd been tempted to pack up Ally and skedaddle out of town, but where would she go? It would have taken months to get set up with another clinic. Months of falling further and further behind financially.

So instead, she'd convinced herself that if she was careful and kept her head down, she'd be able to avoid Dr. Knox Collins. And it had worked. Until now.

"Need some help?" A deep voice came from right behind her, causing her to jump then grab for the coffee mug as her hand knocked against its side.

"What?" she asked, the word ending with a squeak that made her sound like the mouse her sister had always accused her of being. Looking around, she saw that the other staff members had finally left the room. Clearing her throat, she tried again. "I'm sorry, do you need something, Dr. Collins?"

"I just noticed you staring at the screen," he said, his hand waving toward her computer, "and I wondered if you needed help charting something in the delivery record. One of the nurses was just telling me that it was a difficult delivery you and Lori just attended. Sometimes that complicates the charting."

It had been a difficult delivery with the baby being much larger than expected and its face turned up. It had taken everyone working together to get him out. But with Lori, her midwife preceptor beside her, Bree had been in control of the situation. "No. There's no problem."

"Good. I know Lori's your preceptor, but if there's anything I can do, or anything you have a question about, just ask. I know I'm just here temporarily, but I want to help if I can," Knox said before moving back to his own computer.

Once he wasn't looking over her shoulder, Bree's body relaxed, at least a little. He was still too close and his words just made things worse. Because the biggest surprise she'd had since the day they'd first met was that Dr. Knox Collins didn't seem like the coldhearted, self-absorbed man that her sister had made him out to be. He seemed to be truly interested in the patients and the staff at the clinic.

Or was the overly nice doctor he presented to the staff just an act to make people like him? Didn't the man ever wear something besides a smile on his face? Didn't he ever have a bad day? Maybe if you were the only son of mega-rich country music stars you didn't have bad days.

But no matter how nice the man appeared to be, she had to keep her defenses up around him. The last thing she needed was to have him focus that charm of his on her.

"Why? Do you need more members in your fan club?"

she asked, the sarcasm as thick as the butter on a country biscuit.

Had she really just said that?

Way to keep yourself off his radar, Bree.

"I keep getting the feeling that you have something against me. Do you want to talk about it? Clear the air? Is there something I did?" Knox said, the sincerity in his voice setting her teeth to grinding again. Didn't the man ever get mad?

And what would he say if she told him it was definitely something he'd done? He'd gotten her sister pregnant and then ignored her. Bree couldn't blame him for her sister's death—that had been the result of her sister taking a curve around a mountain too fast—but that didn't mean Bree could forgive him for his part in her sister's last days. For not being a man her sister wanted to help raise her daughter.

She knew she couldn't say any of this. Not if she wanted to keep her promise to her sister. And not if she wanted to protect her niece. Instead, she had to find a way to put some distance between them.

"I'm sorry, Dr. Knox. I appreciate your offer to help. It's just been a long day."

The silence in the room was deafening. She knew he wasn't buying her excuse. She'd spent the past three months avoiding him and apparently he had noticed. Had she been that transparent?

"Hey guys, what's up?" Lori asked as she entered the room. Bree released a slow, steadying breath. She'd known from day one that she and Lori were going to make a good team. Though only a few years older than she was, Lori had been with the practice since she had obtained her midwifery certification. She'd taken Bree in as if they'd been friends for a lifetime, and she shared all her experience and knowledge. Lori was someone people knew they could trust the moment they met her. More than once, Bree had started to spill all her secrets with the midwife.

"I'm almost finished with the charting if you want to look it over," Bree said, turning toward the doorway, glad to end the conversation with Knox.

"Sure," Lori said, looking between the two of them, her eyes seeing more than what Bree wanted her to see. Her preceptor was smart and observant.

"I heard that the two of you had a challenging delivery," Knox said, turning his attention to Lori.

"Posterior delivery, but Bree handled it perfectly," Lori said as she took a seat next to Bree. "She's going to make a great midwife."

"I was just telling her that the staff was saying she did great today," Knox said.

"She did," Lori said. "I'm very proud of her."

Bree ducked her head as her cheeks warmed with a blush that would make the freckles on her nose stand out even more.

Where her sister had thrived on the applause and praises of the press and audiences when they were young, it had always made Bree feel uncomfortable and awkward to have others compliment her. It was one of many reasons she had protested when her sister and their agent had decided it was time to take their duet to the next level in the country music scene.

"I still have a lot to learn," Bree said, making herself lift her eyes and look at her coworkers.

"Dr. Collins, they're ready for you in the OR," Kelly, the nurse who'd been giggling with Knox's group earlier, said from the open doorway.

Once Knox left the room, Bree could feel Lori's eyes on her. "What was that about?"

"What?" Bree asked, pretending not to know what Lori was referring to. Unable to hold Lori's gaze, Bree looked back at the computer screen, pretending to study it.

"There was something going on between the two of you. I could feel it."

"It was nothing." All Bree wanted to do was finish her charting and get out of the room before Knox returned.

But the experienced midwife was not going to let it go. Reaching over, Lori shut the door. "I might believe that if this was the first time I'd noticed the change in you when Dr. Collins was around. Has he done something? Anything to make you uncomfortable?"

It seemed that would be the theme of the day. She was too tired to go through another review of all the things Knox had done again.

Still, she knew Lori was concerned that he had done something inappropriate, and Bree couldn't let her think that. "No. He's been nothing but helpful to me since I came to the practice."

"So, what is it, then? I know we were all worried that

he'd be this stuck-up rich kid, but I haven't found him to be that way at all."

Neither had Bree, which had thrown her off, leaving her feeling a guilt that she hadn't expected. Which led her back to the possibility that the man might have truly changed. What if he wasn't the selfish, ego-obsessed man Bree had assumed from her sister's description? And even worse, what if he had never been that man?

No. She wouldn't even consider such a thing. Brittany might not have always been up-front when it came to getting what she wanted, but she never would have made Bree promise to keep her daughter away from her father if she hadn't had a good reason for it. Bree, herself, had looked into his background after Brittany had called her and told her about the baby. Knox Collins had been a troubled teenager who'd been kicked out of more than one private academy. Reports of his partying his way through college were all over the local media.

"Of course, if it's something more personal, I wouldn't blame you. The man is certainly nice to look at. I think half the staff is in lust with him." Lori gave Bree a wicked smile. "It's nothing to be embarrassed about. He's not my type, but I get it."

Bree looked over at Lori. The midwife had a natural beauty that came from her generous smile and kind eyes. "What is your type?"

"I'm not quite sure," Lori said, her eyes looking off into space before returning to Bree. "I'm stuck somewhere between wanting a Mr. Darcy and a Jamie Fraser."

Bree hadn't ever cared much for Mr. Darcy, too stuffy,

but she had watched every season of *Outlander* and couldn't help but think that Knox, with his thick light brown curls that fell almost to his shoulders, would make a great Jamie Fraser.

"Really, Lori, there's nothing like that going on." No matter how good-looking the man was, she would never let herself be attracted to him.

Lori studied her a little too long before finally shaking her head. "Okay, but if there is something that's bothering you, I want you to know you can talk to me. No matter what it's about, but especially if it's something that could affect your work."

Bree bit back words that would spill the secret she had worked so hard to keep for the past eight years. She trusted Lori, she did, but there was too much at stake. If the truth came out about who was Ally's father, Bree could lose the child she loved as her own. Let the other midwife think that Bree was harboring some deep longing for Dr. Collins. Better that than she know the truth.

"If you're good, then, I'm going to let you finish up rounds. We don't have any new labor patients, but there is a day-two postpartum on the floor who needs discharge orders put in. You remember Kristina? It's her third baby. No complications. Just look in on her and make sure she doesn't need anything before discharge. You can meet me back at the office when you're finished."

As soon as Lori had shut the door to the physician's work room, Bree dropped her head to the desk. Why did life have to be so complicated? It had always been her sister who had loved drama. Not Bree. She took in a big breath then let it out, along with all the pent-up stress of the past few minutes, and made herself look on the bright side of things. Dr. Collins had only a few more weeks before his ad-locum contract would be finished and he'd be moving on.

She'd managed for weeks to keep her head down around him. And if luck was on her side, she'd be able to continue to avoid him. But then again, when had luck been on her side?

"I'm not sure I understand," Knox repeated for the third time. "I thought Lori was Bree's preceptor," he said to Dr. Warner.

"I'll still be her preceptor," Lori interjected. "I just think that it would be a good thing for her to get an opportunity to do some work in the county women's clinic. You've been saying you need more volunteers to help. This will work out perfectly," Lori said.

There was something about the way that Lori was looking at him that set his warning bells ringing. It reminded him of the look his momma got when she was about to set him up with her newest matchmaking victim.

"Lori's right," Dr. Warner said as he looked at the two of them from across his desk. "Brianna needs to get some experience in a women's clinic like the one run by the county. There is no telling where she might find herself in the future. Our clinic is lucky enough to have fancy equipment with all the bells and whistles. If she ends up in one of the more rural parts of our state, she might not have those."

Jack was right. The older man had built Legacy Women's Clinic into one of the best clinics in the state during his career. And though he'd stepped back and let his son take over a lot of the running of the clinic now, Knox respected the man and couldn't deny that Jack wanted only the best for all his staff. Unfortunately, that meant Knox was going to have to agree with him. With the shortage of obstetricians nationwide and the rural areas of Tennessee depending on the certified midwives to fill in where they could, Bree would be welcomed in one of the rural areas.

"Okay. Fine. I'll work with her. But I need to know her proficiencies as well as her weaknesses. I don't want to put her in a position she's not comfortable with." It was bad enough that she seemed to have taken to immediately disliking him, something that he still didn't understand. There was even the possibility that Bree would refuse to work with him.

There was a soft knock on the door before Bree stuck her head inside. "You wanted to see me?"

Knox could see the hesitancy in her expression as she entered the room and looked around. When her eyes met his, all the color drained from her face. At that moment she looked so young with her strawberry blond hair pulled back in a tight braid that was a little lopsided. There was an innocence in her green eyes that sparked a sudden, unexpected need to protect her. Just how innocent was she? He hadn't missed the fact that she'd actually blushed when Lori had complimented her earlier that day. When had he ever seen a woman do that? Had he ever?

His attitude concerning Jack and Lori's request to allow the young midwife to work with him at the county clinic made a U-turn. Bree needed to get out into the real world. It had certainly been an eye-opener for him. And one that had changed his whole career. It would be interesting to watch her interact with the women he saw there. Women who didn't have the resources for the kind of care they received at Legacy. Women down on their luck and needing help.

"Come in, Brianna," Jack said, then waved her to the seat next to Knox. "We were just discussing with Dr. Collins the possibility of you helping him out at the county clinic for a few hours a week."

Knox wouldn't have thought her face could have gone any whiter, but it did. For a moment she just stared at Jack, then she turned to Lori. "Is there a problem with me working with you?"

"No, not at all," Lori reassured her. "You are doing beyond what I could have hoped for at this stage of your training. But Jack and I think that you could be an asset to the county clinic while increasing your experience. Here we have a controlled atmosphere where we see our patients on a schedule so we can prepare for our day. At the clinic, you will see more of a variety of patients, including more gynecology patients. It's also something that will look good on your résumé. More importantly, you'll be helping women who need your care."

"I've helped out at Legacy House when I've had the time," Bree said. "And I have…other responsibilities. I don't have a lot of free hours."

"We wouldn't expect you to work any more hours. If Dr. Collins agrees to this, you'll be able to get your clinic hours at the county two days each week in exchange for two days in the clinic here."

When they all turned toward him, Knox felt the tension in the room soar. While Jack's eyes seemed confident that Knox would agree, and Lori had one eyebrow lifted in challenge, Bree's eyes were round as saucers with a fear he could not understand. Had he somehow intimidated her? Was that what all this tension he felt around her was all about? No, the comments she'd made that morning, ones he'd chosen to ignore, showed that she wasn't afraid to speak her mind with him.

Maybe it was because of who his parents were. That, he was used to. A lot of people were overly impressed by his parents' fame. But somehow he knew that wasn't it, either. This was something different. And for some irrational reason, while it should have irritated him, it intrigued him. He wanted to know what it was that had her bristling every time he came into the room.

"I think it would be a great learning experience for Bree, and I could certainly use the help," he said. Neither of those statements was a lie. The clinic was chronically short on staff. He was only filling in for a friend for a few weeks, but he could use the help, even if it was temporary.

Then Bree did something he wasn't expecting. She

pulled back her shoulders and sent all of them a confident, though a little wobbly, smile. "Okay, then. It's settled. I look forward to working with Dr. Collins at the county clinic."

The tremble of her lips as she said the words betrayed that she did everything but look forward to the next month of the two of them working together. Was he the only one in the room who could see she was most definitely not excited about working with him at all? From the smiles on Lori's and Jack's faces, he was afraid that he was.

It had been a long time since he'd had this amount of interest in a woman. Bree Rogers was a mystery, one that he couldn't wait to solve.

"Is this about this morning?" Bree asked as soon as she and Lori were alone in Lori's office.

"Of course not," Lori said and then sighed. "Okay, maybe a little. The truth is Jack mentioned the idea to me and I thought it might be good for you to take this opportunity, not just to learn more about how to work in a county clinic, but also to learn to work with coworkers that you might not like."

"I don't not like Dr. Collins. I just don't..." She'd talked herself into a corner now. How did she explain to Lori her feelings for Knox without spilling all her secrets? "I don't find him particularly likeable."

Lori rolled her eyes at Bree's contradictory statement. "Like I said, Jack—Dr. Warner—came up with this idea. To be honest, I think there's a possibility he has heard some of the office chatter suggesting that you have a problem with Knox. I'm not the only one who has noticed how you have a habit of avoiding our ad-locum doc."

She should have known she couldn't keep her feelings toward the doctor hidden in such a tight-knit group as the one that worked at Legacy Clinic. Did that mean they were talking about her behind her back? Did they, like Lori had, think she had some schoolgirl crush on him?

"Look at it this way. There's only a few more weeks to Dr. Collins's contract here. Do a good job and learn everything you can at the clinic. He's a good doctor. You might be surprised how much he can teach you. He might not have been a doctor for very long, but he's worked some places so far back in the mountains that the nearest hospital was over an hour's drive away."

Bree had heard that Knox had even done some work off the grid up in the Smoky Mountains, which in spite of herself she wanted to hear more about. And like Lori had reminded her, Knox's contract would be over soon and he would be moving on. She just had to hold it together till then. She'd kept her sister's secret for eight years. She could do it a few more weeks.

That thought had her feeling better, until a few hours later when she arrived to pick Ally up from her after-school care program. Seeing her little girl surrounded by her friends as they worked on a craft project made all her protective instincts kick in. Just eight years old, Ally was already showing signs of being a people magnet like her mother. Unlike Bree, who'd been shy most of her childhood, her sister Brittany had always had a way with people. Ally's friendly smile and quick laughter helped her make friends wherever she went. She was sweet and innocent and Bree would protect that little girl with the last breath in her body. She would never allow the man whom her sister didn't approve of take Ally away from her. Never.

"How was your day? Did you deliver any babies?" Ally asked.

Bree flipped a pancake over before turning to her niece. The last thing she wanted to do was talk about her day, but she couldn't ignore the question.

When Ally had started school and Bree had her own classes along with two jobs sometimes, it had become hard for Bree to spend the quality time she wanted to with Ally. Most nights dinner had become fast food or boxed mac-'n'-cheese, so Bree made the effort to make the middle of the week meal fun and a chance for the two of them to spend time together. Since Ally's favorite meal was breakfast, Bree had deemed Wednesday night as breakfast night.

"I did deliver a baby. A really big one with adorable chubby cheeks." Bree turned around and puffed her cheeks out, making a face that had Ally laughing. "What about you? Did the teacher like the picture you drew?"

Ally's laughter stopped and her eyes filled with tears.

"What's wrong? Did something happen to the picture?" While Ally's picture, one that showed Bree and Ally in front of the small house Bree rented, wouldn't have won any awards, she had worked hard on it, and Bree knew Ally's teacher had to have seen that.

"Holly asked me why I didn't have a mommy or daddy," Ally said, before wiping her eyes with her shirt-sleeve.

This wasn't the first time someone in Ally's class had asked her that question. Bree had struggled with the decision of whether to tell Ally about her mother or whether to let her grow up believing that Bree was her mother. To Bree, Ally had been her little girl from the moment the nurse had put her in her arms.

Still, no matter how much Bree loved Ally as her own, it was important that she knew about her mother. In some ways, Ally helped to keep her sister's memory alive for both of them.

Bree knew grief. She and Brittany had lost their parents within a few months of each other. It had been hard, but she'd still had her sister. They'd shared everything from a womb to a room for the first eighteen years of their lives. Not having her sister left a hole that ate at Bree. It was only in the middle of the night, after Ally was safely tucked into bed, that Bree allowed herself to let the grief of losing her sister take over. But the next morning, she pasted on a smile and went back to living, for her sister as much as for her niece.

After taking the pancake from the griddle, Bree went around the island and hugged the little girl. "I'm sorry. I know it makes you sad when someone asks you questions about your mommy."

As always, she avoided the question of Ally's daddy,

something she knew she wouldn't be able to do for too much longer. Till now Ally had been satisfied with Bree's explanation that there had been an accident that had taken her mother away, but it was only a matter of time till the child became more curious about her father. And what was Bree going to do then? She'd found it hard each time she had to explain to Ally how her mother had died; explaining that her father hadn't been in the picture when she'd been born would be even harder.

Ally snuggled closer against her and Bree's arms tightened around her small frame.

For now, all Bree could do was give Ally all the love she had and hope it would be enough to shield her from that and all the other heartbreaks she was bound to encounter. Bree knew she'd always appreciated having her parents to lean on when she'd faced her own heartaches. Of course, that was before the cancer had taken her momma and the bottle had taken her daddy. And then the search for fame had taken Brittany into a whole different place in life than Bree had wanted to go, taking Brittany completely out of Bree's life.

"How about we eat a bunch of pancakes until our tummy hurts and then we can snuggle up together with a couple books till bedtime?"

"Not schoolbooks?" Ally asked. Bree knew she was remembering the months, no, years, that Bree had spent studying for her nursing degree and then her nurse practitioner and midwifery degrees.

"Not schoolbooks," Bree said, though she did have some community health studying she'd planned to do to start preparing for whatever she might encounter with Knox at the clinic. The more she knew, the fewer questions she'd have to ask him.

But later, after their meal and dishes were done, Bree noticed that Ally wasn't paying attention as she read the little girl one of her favorite wizard books. "Do you want us to read something else?"

"I don't feel much like reading. I thought maybe you could tell me a story about my mom instead?"

Bree wasn't surprised at her request after their discussion earlier that night. Bree had been telling Ally stories about Brittany since she was around three. If Bree added a bit to the stories sometimes, it was always for the little girl's benefit. The truth was there were a couple years when Brittany had cut Bree out of her life, which was something Bree would never tell Ally.

"Well, let's see. Where do you want me to start?" Bree asked, though she already knew the answer.

"Start where you and my mom came to Nashville and sang on stage at the Grand Ole Opry," Ally said, snuggling farther down into her covers. "When the two of you were famous."

Bree laughed. "I don't think the two of us were exactly famous. There just weren't a lot of eleven-year-old twins playing guitar and singing Loretta Lynn songs back then."

"Loretta who?" Ally asked.

"Never mind." She'd hold the history of country music lesson till later. "Okay, so you know we'd won a contest at the county fair and made the papers. And then one morning our momma got a phone call inviting us to come sing a couple songs on stage in Nashville. Of course she agreed, but our daddy thought it was a hoax…"

"A what?" Ally asked.

"It's what they used to call scams. Anyway, he called the Opry and asked to speak with the manager, who told him no, it wasn't a hoax. They had seen the article in the paper and they had invited us. It was a good thing it wasn't a scam, too, because our momma was so excited that she had already left the house to pick us up early from school." Bree could still remember the way her momma's eyes had shined when she'd had the principal pull them out of class to tell them. She didn't think she had ever seen her momma so happy. Then Brittany had squealed loud enough that the teachers had stuck their heads out of their classrooms to see what was going on. Before long, the whole school was caught up in the celebration. No one seemed to notice that Bree wasn't celebrating with them. Not even her mother or her sister.

"Tell me about the dress my momma wore," Ally said.

"I've showed you pictures," Bree said, unable to keep the grumble from her voice. She had hated those dresses with the yards of ruffles and bows. The fact that they had been pink, her sister's favorite color, not hers, had nothing to do with it, either. "It was awful. It had all those ruffles and too much lace. It was way too girly."

Ally giggled. "I think it was pretty."

"So there we were, Saturday night, out on the stage, when Loretta Lynn herself came up to your momma and told her that she was 'just the prettiest thing I ever saw.'"

"But you weren't there because you were sick in the dressing room," Ally said.

It had been one of Bree's most embarrassing moments. She'd been throwing up so hard her eyes had watered, and one of the women who worked backstage had to help her clean herself up before she could go on stage. "No, but my momma told me all about it."

"Then the two of you sang that song about being from the country and one of the people there offered y'all a lot of money to sing for them."

"Something like that." Bree was too young to know anything about the money side, but it was the night they got their first agent. Their first in a long line for the next eight years as Brittany and her parents chased their dream for fame and fortune, despite Bree trying to explain to them that she wanted something different for her life.

"I bet if my momma was here right now she'd be a big star. Then I could draw pictures of the three of us up on stage together." Ally yawned and rolled over on to her side, her eyes closing as the long day caught up with her.

"I bet she would," Bree whispered, though in her heart she wasn't so sure. Bree's and Brittany's thirty seconds of fame had been long gone by the time Brittany had died. Brittany had blamed Bree. It had caused a rift between them that Bree had hoped someday to mend. She liked to think that the two of them were moving toward that after the call she received from Brittany before the car crash.

Bree sat there for a few moments until she was sure

that the little girl was asleep, then went to her own room to spend a few hours studying. She had no idea what she might encounter at the county clinic but she was going to be as prepared as possible.

Later, when her eyes refused to read another case study, Bree put her books away and climbed into bed. Somehow, she'd managed to avoid the dreaded conversation about Ally's father once more. But for how long? There was going to come a day when she wouldn't be able to avoid that question. And what was she going to say then? How did she tell a story that she didn't really know herself? All she'd been told by Brittany was that she and Knox had been involved and that he'd left her and had no interest in a child. How did you tell a child that her father hadn't wanted her?

And how did Bree know if that was still the way Knox felt now? Brittany's words had been so cryptic that she wasn't even sure if Brittany had ever told him about the pregnancy. There were so many questions she'd never been able to ask her sister. She was having a hard time believing the man she'd watched interacting with the staff today wouldn't want to know his daughter. And if he did? What would that mean for Ally? For Bree?

Since the moment she'd been told by Dr. Warner and Lori that she would be working with Knox at the clinic, Bree had felt a sense of impending doom. As a midwife, she knew that when a patient felt that way, you never ignored it. There was always some reason, some instinctual knowledge, for that intense feeling that something bad was about to happen.

 Even as she slipped into sleep, she acknowledged that everything in her life was about to change and all she could do was ensure that she protected her niece no matter what it cost her. Because after losing everyone else in her family, she would not lose Ally.

CHAPTER TWO

KNOX WATCHED AS Bree entered the aged county building where the small women's clinic where he was filling in for a friend was located.

"Good morning," he said, startling the young midwife as she reached the top of the first set of stairs that
would lead to their second-floor office. She looked up
at him with her bright green eyes that he always found
appealing. Then there was that long strawberry blond
hair and those freckles that dusted her nose. She wasn't
striking and she didn't fit the trendy idea of beautiful.
What was it about her that kept his mind returning to
her over and over again?

He shook his head at his early-morning musings. He'd
only had time for one cup of coffee so far and it would
take a couple more before he'd be ready for clinic hours.

"I have to say that I'm surprised to find you working
at one of the city's free clinics," Bree said as she looked
around the worn floors and walls that were in deep need
of new paint. She didn't seem to be judging the building
as much as she was judging him.

"I ran into a friend from college who works here and
he needed some time off. The clinic is only open two

days a week. It's not really any different from the work that I do when I'm working up in the mountains. I'd already planned to take the temporary position with Legacy, so why not help him out?"

"I wouldn't think you'd have the time. It almost sounds like you don't do anything but work. Which doesn't make sense."

Knox wasn't surprised by her comment. A lot of people figured that with parents as rich as his, there wasn't any reason for him to work. What they didn't get was that he enjoyed his work. Especially work like he got to do in the rural communities in the mountains. "Both jobs are temporary. And both are very different. You won't see the same clientele here that you've been seeing at the Legacy Clinic. A lot of these women don't have insurance or even money to cover high copays. Some of them don't trust the state health care system. And some of them won't trust you, either. Getting someone to trust you after they've been let down by the system is a major accomplishment. You'll find trust in short supply here. You might not even like the work. It can be very repetitive, mostly yearly exams, medication refills, STD testing, that type of thing. But I can guarantee that it will open your eyes to the needs of the community."

"I'm here to learn as much as possible. Dr. Warner and Lori think this will be good for my training, and their opinions are important to me. I've worked in a labor and delivery department with patients from all backgrounds so that won't be a problem."

This was probably the longest conversation they'd ever

shared. Fortunately for the two of them, there was none of the sarcasm she'd been so happy to share with him the week before, which made him feel better about bringing her in to help out. Maybe having a week to adjust to the idea of working with him had been good, though he still didn't understand what it was about him that caused her to go on the offensive every time she was around him.

"That's good," Knox said as they headed up the second set of steps. He liked the fact that Bree wasn't afraid to stand up and say what she thought. He'd had too many coworkers who treated him differently either because he was a doctor or because of his parents. Bree didn't seem to be impressed by either. "I wanted to show you around the building before we went upstairs to the office since when the doors open I won't have the time. Most of the first story takes care of the county clerk business, but the second floor is mostly used by the health department. At the end of the hall is the children's clinic, which you might need to know to refer some of our patients with children there. And before that, on the right, there is a dentist office and health records departments. There is a substance abuse center across from there. Unfortunately you will need to make referrals there, too."

He watched as she studied the areas he pointed out. When she didn't make any comment, he continued. "Any OB patients get referred out. The health department has a separate program for them."

Turning left, he led her to the set of offices where they'd be working together. The simple block letters that read Women's Clinic was the only thing that set itself apart from the other line of doors down the hall. Opening the door, they were met with the one thing that made the clinic possible, its no-nonsense, but still empathetic, office manager.

"Bree, I'd like you to meet the real boss of this joint, Ms. Lucretia Sweet. Don't be fooled by the name. She's only sweet when she wants to be."

"And I'm certainly not sweet till I get my brew in the morning. Hand it over."

Knox did as he was told and handed the special order coffee to the woman who had won his heart the first day he'd shown up to work there.

"Bree's a midwifery resident at Legacy and is going to be helping for the next few weeks so don't run her off," Knox said. "And if you can show her around while I start a pot of real coffee, I'd appreciate it."

"Me run off good help? Especially when it's free? Not going to happen. Come on in here, Bree. Is that short for Brianna?"

"Yes, ma'am. Brianna Rogers, but please call me Bree."

Knox listened to the women's exchange as he started the coffee in the small corner that also provided snacks and water for their patients. After his first good swallow of the dark-roasted drink, he returned to find Lucretia questioning his resident like a military drill sergeant.

"Have you ever worked in a clinic like this? Because I want you to understand that while we might not agree with some of these women's choices, we treat each one of them as equals."

"I did a rotation in the county jail during my masters in nursing degree. I plan on doing my doctorate dissertation on the need for more women's care in the correctional system."

"I didn't know you were planning on getting your doctorate," Knox said as he leaned against the doorjamb and studied the woman. She was gutsy and driven. He liked that. She'd do well as a midwife wherever she went.

"I'm sure there's a lot you don't know about me," Bree said, then squeezed her lips together as if she wanted to take back the words.

"A woman of mystery. Well, you give me time and I bet I'll learn all those secrets you're keeping," Lucretia said. "Now, let me take you back to the exam offices so I can show you how I set up the supplies. Mind you, don't be wasting them. They don't grow on trees and the budget's tight for this place."

Knowing that Bree was in good hands, he left them to it and went back to top off his cup of coffee. The two women had just met, but already Bree was talking with Lucretia like the two of them were old friends. It seemed she was only prickly with him. So what was it about him that made the woman's back go up every time he was around? Was it because of who his parents were? He'd met a lot of people who were intimidated by his parents' fame, but he still didn't think she was one of them.

The door to their offices opened and he heard Lucretia welcome their first patient of the day. It looked like the mystery of Midwife Bree Rogers would just have to wait.

* * *

By lunchtime, Bree understood immediately why Knox had referred to Lucretia as the boss. From the time the first patient came through the door until when they took a thirty-minute break to swallow down some takeout, the woman had kept the line of patients that filled the small rooms organized and constantly moving.

Lori had told her that she would be starting off working one-on-one with Knox, but by the time they'd seen the first ten patients, Knox had assigned her one of the exam rooms as her own and told her to let him know if she needed him. It had felt good that he had confidence in her skills, even if she shouldn't have cared what he thought. Since then, she'd seen another six patients on her own and after figuring out the computer system for ordering lab tests and pharmacy prescriptions, she'd not had any trouble. She'd discovered quickly that most of the women the clinic saw were young and seeking an inexpensive way to obtain birth control or to be tested for STDs or pregnancy, all things that she'd been well trained in at the Legacy Clinic, though she'd quickly learned that giving these women a prescription didn't always mean the women could afford it.

When one woman she saw explained that the reason she had returned after being seen the month before was that she couldn't afford to get the birth control prescription filled, Bree had gone into the storage closet and taken out a six-month supply for the woman, along with a handful of condoms that she stuffed into the bag before the woman had left. The look on Lucretia's face when the woman walked out told Bree that the boss knew exactly what she had done and would be watching her. Giving the *boss* a guilty wave, Bree had slinked back into her assigned exam room to see her next patient. Yes, she knew they were working on a limited supply of samples of medication, but how much more wasteful would it be if the woman had to return every month? It would still be the same amount of samples given.

By the time they had stopped for their break, she was prepared to support her argument in case she was called on the carpet by either Lucretia or Knox.

"So, any issues?" Knox asked her as he handed her a canned drink and sandwich.

"No, it's all been good," she said, looking over at Lucretia. When the woman didn't say anything to the contrary, Bree figured she'd been worrying for nothing.

"I know this work isn't as exciting as delivering babies, but some of the women who come here have no place else to turn for basic care. My friend Dean, who runs this place, spends almost as much time working to get financing for supplies as he does seeing patients. I don't know exactly what his salary is, but if it's anything like what I receive when I'm working out in the small rural areas, it isn't much."

She'd only been working there a few hours, but already she could see that there was a true need in the community. How could one clinic that was only open two days a week provide for the needs of a city the size of Nashville?

"If you like the work, I know he would be happy to have the extra help," Knox said.

"I don't know what I'm going to do when I finish my residency. I have to pass my boards and then…" Had she really been about to say she had a little girl to take care of? "I just have a lot on my plate."

"I understand," Knox said, shrugging, before looking away. Bree had a strange feeling that she had disappointed him somehow.

"I'm sorry. I just can't commit to anything right now. I've been going nonstop for several years now and… I have other responsibilities that I need to take care of."

"It's okay, Bree. I didn't mean to put you on the spot. I just noticed that you seemed to be enjoying the job, and the patients seemed to be comfortable with you. But then I hear you've always been great with the patients at the clinic. You know I've helped start clinics like this one in the rural mountain towns where I've worked. I've even left some of them with a midwife in charge."

"Really?" she asked. "I'm surprised you could do that."

"The state of Tennessee allows midwives to work on their own without a doctor present. Of course, they all have doctors as resources and can refer out as needed. And not all the clinic services are free. If a patient has insurance, the clinic can file for reimbursement. A lot of their patients do have funding, they just don't have anywhere to go without traveling more than an hour."

"That sounds like an interesting job," Bree said. She could imagine herself living in a rural area someday.

A place where Ally would have plenty of room to run and play.

"If you ever decide you're interested, get in contact with me. After watching you today, I think you might enjoy the work," Knox said.

Bree could feel the blush creep up her face with the compliment. Why did this man have to keep being so nice to her? She didn't want him to be nice. She wanted him to be...well, she didn't know what she wanted him to be, but she didn't want him to be like this. His being nice just increased the guilt and fear she had that everything she'd believed about him wasn't true. And that wasn't something she could consider.

Because if you've been wrong all this time, if this man would have been a proper parent for Ally, how are you going to live with the fact that you didn't contact him after Brittany's death? And what do you do about Ally then? Can you live with the guilt that you knew he was Ally's father and never told him? Or her?

It had been easy to keep silent about Ally when her father had been some undeserving sperm donor. But now, actually getting to know the man herself, she couldn't conceive that the man her sister had made sound so cold and uncaring was the same man sitting across from her. The same man who went across the country starting clinics for underserved communities.

And it wasn't just that she had taken Brittany's word. Bree had done some investigating herself. There was no doubt that Knox had gotten into trouble during his teenage years. It had been small things, but she knew those things usually grew to bigger things when a teenager got older. There were also reports of him going to rehab more than once. Had he really changed his life that much? From everything she had seen since meeting him, it seemed that he had.

Bree's hands began to shake as she lifted the sandwich toward her mouth. Her stomach protested at the thought of taking another bite. What was she going to do? Tell him about Ally? She'd promised her sister that she would keep her secret. How could she ignore her sister's last request?

"Are you okay?" Knox's hand reached out across the table, just stopping before it covered hers. "You look a little pale."

Looking up, her eyes met his and she bit back a groan when she saw the concern there. "I'm fine. I'm just tired."

Her eyes remained locked on his and the guilt she'd felt earlier changed to something more disturbing. As she realized how close the two of them were, her unsteady stomach suddenly seemed to be filled with happy little butterflies performing an unfamiliar dance. Looking down, she saw his hand, strong and steady, so close to her own. She was shocked to find that she wanted to reach out her own hand and cover his. She wanted to feel that connection of skin to skin. She wanted to feel the warmth of his fingers slipping over hers. She wanted to find some comfort from this mess she'd made and the consequences she had to face.

"I hate to hear that," Lucretia said from the doorway, causing the both of them to jump, "because I've got a pregnant woman that just walked in saying she's having contractions, and I don't know nothing about delivering babies."

The two of them jumped up, with Knox beating her to the front of the office where a woman who looked not far from a full-term pregnancy was bent over at the waist.

"I tried to get her to sit down, but she won't budge," Lucretia said.

Even with her limited experience, Bree could see the woman was deep into laboring. She and Knox looked at each other. Gone was the intimacy she'd felt before. They were back to business. Thank goodness.

"Lucretia, call 911 and tell them we have a woman in labor," Knox said.

"What's your name?" Bree asked, putting her arm under the woman's to help support her when her pregnant body relaxed in relief as the contraction ended.

"Elena," the woman said, her dark brown eyes looking up at Bree. "My name is Elena. The pain, it's so hard."

"It's okay. There's an ambulance coming that will take you to the hospital where they can help with that. How many weeks are you?" Knox asked as he looped his arm around the woman's other side.

"The baby...he is due next month," the woman gasped out as another contraction started.

Half lifting, half dragging, they helped the woman into the first exam room, pausing when another contraction hit, causing her to double over with the pain.

Bree squatted down in front of her and took her hands. "Breathe with me. It will help."

Eyes drowning with the pain met Bree's, searching for help. "Let's get you up on the exam table so Dr. Collins can check to see how dilated you are."

Knox lifted the woman up while she gripped Bree's hand with a strength that seemed inhuman.

"Next contraction, we'll breathe together." As the next contraction hit, Bree coached the woman into deep breathing through it, Bree's eyes demanding the woman's dark brown ones to focus on her, as Lucretia and Knox helped set up for examination. "That was great. You are doing so good. You said the baby was a boy?"

"A boy, yes. A son," Elena said.

"The contractions are less than two minutes apart. That ambulance better get here fast," she said to Knox before another contraction hit her patient.

"Look at me," she told Elena, trying to keep the woman's focus centered on breathing.

"I don't think it's going to matter how fast the ambulance goes," Knox said. "Lucretia, get me some blankets and the emergency box."

Knox's words and the worried look in his eyes told her that something was wrong. As he mouthed the word *feet*, Bree's heart rate spiked and her hand tightened on the young woman's. A footling breech delivery was difficult and dangerous in the best of settings. Here? Where they had no anesthesia, no NICU nurses, no option except to deliver vaginally? This was the worst possible situation.

Lucretia rushed into the room carrying a box labeled emergency delivery and a stack of white hospital blankets.

"Elena, your baby is coming, but he's coming out with

his feet first. I'm going to need you to listen closely to Dr. Collins so we can get him out safely. Can you do that for me?"

Elena nodded her head, fear replacing the pain in her eyes. Bree wanted to watch Knox work, to see what was happening. There were so many things that could go wrong. A prolapsed cord. Entrapment. Elena's baby was in real danger, but Bree knew she couldn't let her worry show. It was too important that Elena stayed in control. It could determine the baby's survival.

"Okay, Elena, you're going to feel a lot of pressure. I need to maneuver the baby the rest of the way out, but I don't want you to push. Just pay attention to Bree. She'll help you."

Bree's hands tightened on Elena's while placing her face inches from the other woman's. "You've got this, Elena."

"But the pressure…" Elena's voice broke on a groan.

"Look at me. You are going to pant with me now," Bree said, using her momma voice that told Ally she had better be listening to her. Elena's eyes returned to her and the two of them began to pant, their sounds filling the room.

"Come on, little guy, help me out here," Knox said, before Elena gasped, then collapsed back on the exam table.

"He's out!" Lucretia shouted from the end of the exam table as the sound of a faint cry, followed by a very loud, pissed-off wail, filled the room.

"He's okay," Elena said. "He's really okay?"

"He's fine," Knox said, holding up the screaming baby. Bree noticed that the baby was on the small side, but his color was turning a beautiful, healthy pink with his crying.

Her eyes met Knox's and at that moment something passed between them as they shared the joy of a new life coming into the world; something unlike anything she had ever experienced. It was as if pieces of a puzzle slid into place, bonding them together right then and there. She didn't want to look away, knowing that she would lose this shared moment when she did.

Voices came from the office entrance. The ambulance had finally arrived.

Minutes later Elena, with her son held tightly in her arms, was loaded up on the stretcher for their trip to the hospital. As soon as they left the exam room, Knox sank to the floor, his back pressed up against the exam table. Unable to stop herself, Bree followed him down.

"I was so afraid you wouldn't be able to get him out in time," she said.

"Me, too," Knox admitted, removing the gloves he still wore and dropping them on the floor. The room was a mess, but cleaning it could wait.

"I couldn't tell. You seemed so calm."

"We were lucky that the baby was small and it wasn't her first. The fact that we didn't have a prolapsed cord was a miracle. I don't know what I would have done if you hadn't been there to keep Elena in control. You were great with her. We made a great team, didn't we?"

"We did," she said.

Bree liked the fact that he included her, making her feel as if her part in helping to get the little one out was just as important as his.

"I'm a likeable guy, if you give me a chance."

Bree was afraid he was right. Even though she didn't want to admit it.

Lucretia rushed back into the room and stopped, seeing the two of them on the floor together. "What do y'all think you're doing? If you think the two of you are just going to lie around for the rest of the day, you better start thinking again. We've got a hallway of women waiting for me to open the door. We ain't got no time for the two of you peacocking around because y'all delivered a baby."

Turning, the woman headed out the door, calling back, "You got two minutes, then I'm letting in the horde."

"You're a tough taskmaster, Lucretia," Knox called after her.

"And if you make me stay after five you'll be paying me overtime," the woman called back.

The two of them looked at each other and Bree realized just how close they sat together. Close enough for her to see that there were little flecks of brown scattered throughout his light gray eyes that seemed to match the light brown hair that curled around his face. Her breath caught. He was a beautiful-looking man. She looked away, hoping he hadn't noticed her staring at him.

"I guess we had better get back to work," Knox said, standing and then offering her a hand.

Bree looked at the hand he held out. Something had

changed between the two of them over the past few minutes. Working together to deliver Elena's baby had torn more chunks out of the wall of bitterness she had constructed to keep Ally and her safe from him, creating even more confusion inside her. A part of her wanted to build back those walls, to hold on to the anger and bitterness that Brittany had passed on to her. She needed to ignore everything she was beginning to learn about him. The other part of her knew she had to discover the truth. Was he really the kind, caring man he appeared to be? Had he changed so much from the man Brittany had described to her? How was she supposed to discover the real Knox Collins? Maybe working with him was a good idea after all. Maybe it was time she gave him a chance to prove that he could be a good father to Ally.

Looking back at his hand, they both knew that if she took it she would be acknowledging that things had changed between the two of them. Somehow, she knew there would never be any going back after this.

Swallowing down the fear of where accepting the friendship he offered would take her and how that could affect her and her niece's lives, Bree reached for his hand.

CHAPTER THREE

KNOX HAD JUST gotten home when his phone rang. Some
part of him, some crazy part he needed to ignore, had
hoped that it was Bree calling. Instead, he saw that it
was his mother making her daily check in with him.
Why his mom felt the need to make sure he was taking
care of himself now, he didn't know, though he couldn't
deny that a part of him still craved his mother's attention.
Still, he'd tried to explain to her that he was a grown man
who didn't need his mommy checking on him every day.
She'd pushed back, telling him that if he had a wife she
wouldn't feel the need to call every day. He'd dropped
the argument, knowing he'd been outmaneuvered. His
mother was an expert at that. They both knew that there
had been a time when his parents had been so busy with
their country music careers, that they hadn't given him
the time or the supervision he'd needed. It wasn't a co-
incidence that the daily calls had started after his best
friend had died from a car accident that he could easily have been in. Thad's death had affected all of them.

"Hi, Mom," he said as he opened the door to the
fridge.

"Hello, darling, how was your day at the clinic?" His

mother's voice warmed that part of him that went cold with memories of his friend.

"Interesting and very unexpected," he answered. "We delivered a baby on our lunch break."

"A baby? At the clinic? I thought this was a community clinic, not an OB clinic."

"Well, today we changed the rules." Knox stared inside the fridge. What was it he had been looking for?

"We? You mean the manager you told me about helped? I hope she wasn't traumatized. That's not what she signed up for, I'm sure."

"It was unexpected for all of us, but no. I meant the midwife who was working with me." Knox grabbed a bottle of water and shut the refrigerator door. "It was a difficult delivery. I don't know what I would have done if Bree hadn't been there to help keep the mother in control."

"You didn't tell me you had more staff. Tell me more about this Bree. Is she married?" The hopefulness in his mother's voice set off all his warning bells.

"No. At least I don't think so." Bree didn't really talk much about anything outside of work, at least not around him. But there hadn't been a ring on her finger. He knew because he'd checked not long after they had met. Not that it had done any good. It had only taken a couple of weeks at the Legacy Clinic for him to realize the woman did not care for him at all. And that was putting it mildly. She'd shut him down the first conversation he'd tried to start with her, and things had only gone down from there.

"What's wrong? Is it this Bree woman?" his mother

asked. He wondered sometimes why scientists hadn't been able to discover just where a mother's intuition was located. He had no doubt that it did exist.

"I don't understand her at all," Knox said before realizing the giant hole he'd left open for his mother's inquisition.

"Imagine, a man that doesn't understand a woman. I take it this isn't a work thing. You said she helped you with the delivery?"

Knox thought about the way she'd eyed his hand before she'd reached out to him. It had been just a friendly gesture, one that he would have offered to anyone. But with Bree, the way she'd studied it, it had felt like more. And then there'd been the feel of her hand in his. There'd been nothing friendly about the way his heart rate had spiked from the touch of her soft hand sliding inside his. If he'd held on for just a second too long, he didn't think she had noticed.

"No, not exactly work, it's just…" Knox didn't know how to describe the way Bree had reacted to him from day one. "She acts like I've done something to make her mad at me. Or as if somehow I've let her down. But it doesn't make sense. I'd never met her before I started working at Legacy."

"Are you sure of that?" his mother asked. "Women tend to remember more when it comes to, let's say, romantic interludes."

There had been a time when he'd been wild and reckless, and there were a lot of women who had come and gone in those days. But none of them had been Bree.

He was sure of that. He'd remember her. Besides, Bree wasn't the kind of woman who ran after the town's bad boy that he'd been then. She was smarter than that.

"I'm sure. Don't worry about it. It could all be my imagination," Knox said, though he knew it wasn't. "Tell me about Dad. Is he still obsessed with his new golf clubs?"

As his mother talked about his father's golf swing, as well as the new putting green he was insisting they have put in, Knox found himself thinking again about the way Bree had sat so still as she'd studied the hand he'd held out to her, as if she feared taking his offer of help. But it had been more and he'd known it. He'd been extending a hand in friendship.

And even though she'd taken his hand and he knew something had changed between the two of them after working together in the clinic, he couldn't help but think whatever it was she was holding against him was going to come out eventually.

Bree turned around as her name was called from across the bar. Waving to a customer she'd been dodging for the past fifteen minutes, she shouted over the noisy crowd, "I'll be right there."

Was the place exceptionally loud tonight, or was it just that she was getting too old for the job? There was a time, when she was young and just beginning college, that working at The Dusty Jug in downtown Nashville on a Friday night had been the perfect job. Now, after ten years of slinging beers and dealing with the occasionally rowdy tourist, she could do the job on autopilot, something that she found herself doing more and more lately. Being a single mom, a midwife resident and fill-in bar staff was getting to be too much for her. The lack of sleep was beginning to wear on her.

But what were her options? She had food, rent and childcare to pay for and the tips at the bar were good on weekends. If she could just hold on for a few more months, she'd be able to have a normal schedule. Well, as normal as a midwife's schedule could be.

"Is that guy bothering you?" Mack asked from behind the bar.

"He's just another guy who's partied a little too much this weekend. I can handle him." Bree had been handling men like him for years now. The best way to deal with him was to serve him his beer with a smile, then walk away as fast as she could. The place was so busy tonight that she wouldn't have to worry about him following her through the crowd.

Bree delivered an order, then went over to the table where the man who'd waved her down sat with three of his friends, all of them in different states of inebriation. She'd bet her tip money on the three of them being college students who were celebrating the end of the semester. They'd all regret it in the morning, but there wouldn't be any convincing them of that tonight. "What can I get you?"

"How about your number?" the young man asked, then elbowed his friend when he started to laugh.

"Sorry, not tonight," she said. "But I will give you the

number to a car service as there is no way any of you are driving home tonight."

"I've got one," one of the other men stated, waving his phone up in the air toward her.

"Okay, then," she said, turning to leave, only to have the one closest to her grab her arm.

"One more round?" he asked, giving her a smile that made him look even younger.

She looked down at his hand pointedly, and he immediately let go.

"Sorry, ma'am," he said, his eyes dropping from hers.

"One more, then you call for a ride," she said, then pointed over to Danny, the bouncer on duty. "I'm telling him to keep an eye on y'all and make sure you get a safe ride home. No more bars, either. You all go home."

All four heads turned toward the man standing at the door. Six feet five and over two hundred fifty pounds, Danny had played offense for the Vanderbilt Commodores back in his college days and now coached football at one of the local high schools. He was all muscle, and wearing a skintight T-shirt, he proved he was not afraid to show it off. Anyone who thought they'd act out at the Dusty Jug changed their mind when Danny looked their way.

Heading back to the bar for their order, she was stopped when Sara, one of the other waitresses, flagged her down. "Mack said the band is running fifteen minutes late and he wants you to cover for them."

"That's the third time this month. Mack needs to do something about them." It wasn't that Bree minded entertaining the crowd. She'd been doing it for years and Mack would make sure the band gave her a share of their tips. And even when the bar was busy like tonight, it wasn't the same as getting up on a concert stage where those huge blinding lights kept you from seeing the people you were supposed to be performing for. "Can you take care of the group at table twenty? Tell Mack they only get one more round, he knows what they're drinking, and then they're out of here."

"Got it," Sara said, rushing back to the bar.

After stopping to give Danny a heads-up on the group of young men in case they tried to sneak past the bouncer, she headed back to the staff lounge where she kept her guitar stashed for times like this. She stopped by a mirror and couldn't help but remember that first time she'd gone on stage, dressed up in that ridiculous pink dress, with her sister beside her. Life hadn't turned out the way any of them had expected then. Her dreams and her sister's had been so different. Her sister loved the stage from the moment they'd walked out in front of those glaring spotlights, while Bree had only wanted to run off stage and hide in their dressing room until it was all over.

She couldn't help but ask herself if things would have been different for Brittany if Bree had just gone along with her sister's plans. Yes, Bree wouldn't have been happy with a life in the spotlight. But would that have been so bad if it meant she would still have her sister?

Thinking about Brittany as she climbed up on the small platform that acted as the bar's stage, Bree ran her fingers over the guitar strings, making adjustments before picking out a song she'd written one night after her sister had died. She'd never sung it in public, it wasn't a bar kind of song, but when her fingers played the intro to the song she had written so long ago, she began to sing.

Knox hadn't been crazy about a night of bar hopping. He'd left that scene years ago and had never looked back. But it was his cousin's bachelor party; his attendance had been demanded. Now, after two hours of going from one overcrowded bar to another, he was already planning his escape. He'd spent too much of the first years of his college life at bars, something he was still trying to live down. With his reputation as a doctor always on the line, he was now aware of everything he did. He never wanted to be thought of as Nashville's rebellious bad boy again.

As he followed his cousin and his friends into the next bar on their list, he felt a change in the atmosphere. The Dusty Jug was packed, but instead of the normal rowdy crowd of the other bars, the place was almost silent except for the voice of a young woman singing. Unable to see the stage from where he stood at the entrance, he weaved his way through the crowd, drawn by a voice so sweet and pure, yet for some reason familiar.

Finding a place against the bar, he craned his neck to the side to see a young woman with a guitar in her arms, playing a song whose words spoke of a deep pain of loss. Just the sound of her voice made you want to weep.

"You left me with an angel to heal my heart." The woman sang the chorus, then started on another verse. "When you got your wings, you left an angel with your eyes, your laugh. You left an angel so that I'd always have you with me. As long as your little angel is with me, I'll always have an angel to heal my heart."

As the woman played the last notes then looked up at the crowd, Knox's breath seized in his lungs, his heart stuttering from shock. The crowd's enthusiastic cheers jerked him back to reality and he sucked in a breath. Sitting on the stage, Bree Rogers smiled and thanked everyone before standing as a group of musicians began to take the stage.

Her hair was pulled back into a ponytail, the same way she wore it at work. But with her white T-shirt, cutoff jean shorts and white tennis shoes, she looked too young to even be allowed in the bar, let alone old enough to be delivering babies.

Then he remembered the pain he'd seen in her eyes as she sang. A pain he knew spoke of a heartache she was definitely too young to have experienced. He recognized that pain. It was the pain of loss. He had carried the weight of that pain since the unnecessary death of his best friend. It had been almost nine years and it hadn't gotten any easier.

He watched as she moved toward the bar, then stopped when she spotted him. For a few seconds neither of them moved. None of this made sense. What was the midwife doing here entertaining a bar crowd? He'd never heard anything about her being able to sing like that, either. Not that there weren't thousands of people who had come to Nashville to get a break into the country music world. But he couldn't believe Bree was one of them. Just the little bit he'd worked with her proved that her dedication was to midwifery.

"What are you doing here?" she asked, suspicion in her eyes. Did she think he was stalking her?

"Bachelor party," he said. "What about you?"

She looked down at the T-shirt she wore that displayed the bar's name. "It should be pretty obvious that I work here."

She moved past him and said something to the bartender before turning back to him. "I've got to get back to work. Enjoy your party."

He watched as she walked off, her head held high as she balanced a tray of drinks. He spotted his group at the back of the bar where they'd managed to find a table and went to join them. The mystery of Brianna Rogers just kept getting bigger and bigger. He knew he should let it go. Bree deserved her privacy. But he couldn't seem to do it. The more he learned about her, the more he wanted to know.

It wasn't that hard to figure out that she had to be working at the bar to pay the bills. He didn't know anything about her past. He'd had rich parents to support him while he was in school; most students didn't. But the music, the voice, that was the surprise. Instead of waiting tables, she could have been singing anywhere in Nashville with that voice.

"I saw you talking to that waitress. You know her?" his cousin said, leaning over toward Knox while the other men were busy with a conversation about their golf game that day.

"I thought I did, but now I'm not so sure." But he would. Somehow, someway, he would find out everything there was to know about Brianna. Then maybe this obsession with her would end.

He studied the drink in front of him, refusing to let her catch him studying her. He didn't want her to think he really was stalking her. She might not have accused him of it, but the look she'd given him had spoken of a mistrust. Was it possible that she had a history of being stalked? That would explain a lot about her behavior, not only here, but also at the office. Maybe a bad experience had her keeping her distance from all men.

"I don't know what the two of you have going on, but some guy over there seems to be giving her a hard time," his cousin said, starting to stand.

Knox looked up and saw a young man slam his empty drink glass down on the table then stand. Knox put a hand on his cousin's shoulder and pushed him back into the chair before standing. "Your momma will kick my butt if you get in a bar fight and mess up your pretty face tonight. I've got this."

Most of the crowd was settled around the stage where the band played, making it easy for Knox to cross the room to where Bree was arguing with a kid who had plainly drunk more than he should. He looked over to where the bouncer on duty was busy dealing with three other guys about the same age. They all looked like they were about to fall over. Knox could still remember those days of being old enough to drink legally, but not smart enough to know when to stop.

"Is there a problem?" he asked as he approached. With Bree's hands on her hips and her eyes shooting fire, Knox was glad he wasn't the one in her sights.

Without looking at him, Bree waved him away. "Cooper doesn't want to leave with his friends. For some reason, he thinks I have to serve him a drink even though I've already told him he was cut off."

Knox took in the relaxed way she stood. She wasn't really intimidated by this guy. She was just looking out for the kid and he was too drunk to see it. "Well, Cooper, it sounds like it's time to thank your waitress for her service, leave a big tip for her trouble and head home before you do something that you'll regret in the morning."

When the boy turned, swinging wildly, Knox's arms came up instinctively while he moved himself in front of Bree. The boy's swing met air and the rest of his body followed through, sending him sprawling on to the bar floor.

The sound of Bree's whistle carried over the band and both the bartender and the bouncer headed their way. Within minutes, the kid was off the floor and headed outside with the bouncer, who had assured Knox that the kid and his friends would be tucked into a car from a local service.

"Are you okay?" he asked Bree, once the bar doors closed behind the bouncer.

"I'm fine. I've seen worse," Bree said, then glanced up from where she was gathering empty glasses from the table. "How about you?"

"Unfortunately, I've seen worse, too.' He tried to keep

his voice calm, but he couldn't help but think about the night he and Thad had been out drinking in a bar not much different than this one. Who knows, they might have come to this bar that night. They'd both been too young and dumb to know when they'd reached their limit then. Maybe if someone like Bree had stopped Thad from stumbling outside and getting into his car, his friend would still be here. It had only been the fact that Knox had run into a group from his parents' band that had saved him from joining his friend.

"You sure you're okay?" Bree asked. She'd moved in front of him, dipping her head down until her eyes met his. There was worry in her eyes now. Worry for him.

"Sorry, just memories from long ago when me and my friends thought we knew everything, too," he said. She moved back from him and picked up her tray that she'd loaded with glasses. She started to walk away, back toward the bar, and he tried to find a reason to stop her. "Thank you for looking out for that kid. I wish there'd been someone like you that night."

Turning, she gave him a quizzical look. "What night?"

They stood there, standing in the middle of a bar, and for some reason Knox couldn't stop himself from spilling his guts. "Me and my friend went out partying one night, though we should have been back at the dorm studying for exams. Thad said we'd cram the next day. I was young and stupid. I had dreams of medical school, but I was messing them up. I agreed with him. There was plenty of time for studying. I didn't even try to talk him out of going out. I'd spent most of that year partying instead of studying. I still don't know how I graduated that year."

"What happened?" she asked.

Knox looked around, before looking up at Bree. "You had to have heard all the reports of the wild son of Charles and Gail Collins."

From high school to the day Thad had died, he'd given his parents nothing but trouble. All in the name of a "good time." Back then, if there was a bar fight in downtown Nashville, he had probably been in it. That had been what he thought was a good time.

He didn't want to think about those times. He didn't want to remember that last night when Thad had thrown his arm over Knox's shoulder and told him he'd see him the next day. He didn't want to think about letting his friend walk out, knowing that his friend was as drunk as he was, and never making a move to stop him.

"I let my best friend, as drunk as those kids who just left, walk out of the bar, knowing that he was going to drive himself home. He never made it there."

He saw the shock in her eyes, then the pity that followed. He didn't need her pity. Didn't deserve it.

"Anyway, thanks for watching out for guys like Cooper. I hope someday he realizes he owes you a thank-you." Knox turned and walked back to the table where he could see his cousin's friends were finishing their drinks and getting ready to move on.

He felt raw from the memories and irritated at himself for letting his guard down in front of Bree. He was Dr. Collins now. Her mentor. She needed to trust his guidance. He didn't need to dig up all his past sins for her to see. He'd fought too hard to turn his life around. His memories were of a past he had tried to bury. So why did it feel so important that he share them with Bree?

CHAPTER FOUR

WHEN BREE WOKE up Tuesday morning, she was surprised to find that she was looking forward to a day at the community clinic. Not that she didn't still have reservations about working with Knox; after their conversation at the bar she was more confused than ever. No matter how much she wanted to ignore it, the Knox Collins she was getting to know was not the same one that her sister had known.

But how could someone change that much? Oh, she could understand that Knox had changed his ways as far as being totally centered on partying while he was in college. A lot of kids went down that road before waking up and discovering life wasn't all partying. Bree had no doubt that her sister had been right there in the partying crowd. It was probably where Brittany had met Knox. But there was something else that bothered her. Bree knew Brittany's thirst for fame had always been her sister's driving force. She'd always wondered if Brittany had really just run across Knox at a bar one night, or had she sought him out knowing that Knox's parents could help her in her drive for her career? It was a terrible thing to think about her sister, but Bree had personally seen the things Brittany would do for her career. She had to be honest with herself.

But did it really matter what Brittany's reasons were? Her sister was gone. It was only Ally who mattered now. Her niece would someday look at her and ask about her daddy. And what was Bree to say then? That she'd promised Ally's mother that she'd never tell her father about her? Was it really fair to the child for Bree to hold back information that would affect her whole life? Was it fair to Knox? She knew the answer to both questions. She knew she had to do the right thing for both Ally and Knox. She just didn't know if she had the courage to do it.

Bree was still struggling with her thoughts when she walked into the clinic and was greeted by Lucretia.

"Well, what are you doing coming in here looking like your best friend just died?" Lucretia asked when Bree entered the office with none of the excitement she'd felt that morning. Instead, she felt the weight of years of keeping a secret that she never should have been forced to keep.

"What's wrong?" Lucretia asked, all her teasing gone now.

Bree's mouth refused to move as her throat tightened and her eyes began to water. She looked around the room, beginning to panic. The last thing she needed was for Knox to find her having a meltdown in the waiting room.

"Come on," Lucretia said, then gestured for Bree to follow her back into one of the exam rooms.

"Sit. You've got five minutes to tell me what's wrong.

I can't have you bringing problems here that might affect your work," the woman said as she pointed to an old plastic chair against the back wall. While the woman's words could have seemed cold, her eyes were full of concern.

Bree looked at the chair then back at Lucretia, who stood against the door and Bree's only escape. At that moment Bree realized why she'd come to like the woman so much. Lucretia's take-charge attitude reminded her of her momma's. But while her momma had become blinded by the glitz of the country music world and her dreams for Bree's and Brittany's music career, Lucretia was only looking out for her and the patients at the clinic.

"It's nothing. I'm here to work. I just have some things on my mind." Even as she spoke the words, she wished she could say more. She'd kept her sister's secret for so long. And for what? Everything her sister said wasn't true now, which left Bree with a terrible burden that she didn't think she could carry any longer. "I've done something, something that I thought was the right thing at the time. I kept a secret that I shouldn't have. Now I think I was wrong. Now I have some hard decisions to make because what I've done has affected other people's lives."

Bree swallowed, then forced herself to continue. "And the truth is I'm afraid."

There. She'd said the two words she'd refused to admit even to herself. She was afraid. Afraid of breaking a sacred promise she'd made to her sister just days before Brittany had been killed. Afraid of confronting Knox with the news that he had a daughter. Afraid of telling Ally that she'd had a father her whole life who didn't know about her. But most of all, she was afraid of losing a child that was as much hers as she was Brittany's and Knox's. Whether it had been the right thing to do or not, Bree had raised Ally as her child. And the thought of losing her scared her most of all.

Looking up, Bree saw Lucretia's eyes soften. "Girl, being afraid is part of living. And sometimes it's part of doing the right thing. We don't know each other that well, but I don't think you would have done something to hurt someone. At least, not on purpose."

Bree shook her head. "Just because it wasn't on purpose doesn't mean it won't hurt them."

"Which will hurt them more? Admitting to them that you made a mistake? Or continuing to keep a secret they have the right to know?"

Bree knew the answer to Lucretia's question. She'd already made the decision that she had to tell both Ally and Knox the secret she'd promised never to tell. She had to do the right thing by both of them. Now she just had to figure out how.

"Lucretia? Bree?" Knox's voice called from down the hall. "Where is everybody?"

Bree knew that there was no way that Lucretia could know that her secret involved Knox, but the sound of his voice sent warning signals to her brain while at the same time she felt the heavy weight of guilt in her chest. "Please don't mention any of this to him."

"Anything I hear in these office walls is privileged information, isn't it?" Lucretia asked, then winked at her before the exam door opened and Knox stuck his head inside.

"Is there an office meeting I wasn't notified of?" Knox asked, his voice light and teasing.

"No," Bree said, rushing past the two of them to escape. In a matter of minutes, Lucretia had helped her narrow down the answer to her problem to the simplest of answers. She had to do the right thing, no matter how scared she was.

But first, she had to come up with a plan. It wasn't every day that a man learned he had an eight-year-old daughter. Would he be happy? Angry? He'd certainly be angry that Brittany, and then Bree, hadn't told him about the pregnancy, because the more she got to know Knox, the more she was convinced that he had never known about Brittany's pregnancy. She could understand that he'd be angry with her and she deserved his anger. But no matter how angry he was, they would still have to work together. And they'd have to figure out a way to tell Ally.

They'd have to do that together, too, she decided as she went into the second exam room, pretending to organize the supplies, though she had no doubt Lucretia had seen to that earlier.

Finally, the first patient arrived and her busy day began. Putting her personal problems aside, she focused all of her energy on her patients. Avoiding Knox wasn't a problem. The two of them were kept too busy to even stop for a break.

After seeing twice the number of patients that she

saw in a day at the Legacy Clinic, she'd thought her day over when Lucretia found her in one of the exam rooms setting up for their next clinic day. "There's a girl, she can't be eighteen, that has been pacing outside the office for the last thirty minutes. I tried to talk to her, but she ran off. Now she's back. Can you talk to her and see what she needs?"

Looking at her watch, Bree saw that she was due to pick up Ally in less than an hour. She couldn't be late getting there, again. It seemed she never had enough time anymore.

Both she and Knox were scheduled at the Legacy Clinic the next day, as Lori had rearranged Bree's office and call schedule around Knox's so that Bree could continue to work with her two days a week. And while Bree was happy that she was getting the experience she needed, it was getting harder and harder for her to manage her work at the two clinics, her job at the Dusty Jug and make sure Ally was given the attention she needed.

"She looks scared, Bree. And she's very skittish. I don't want to scare her away again." Bree had only known the office manager for a couple days, but she had already learned to trust Lucretia's instincts.

"I'll try to talk to her. Maybe I can get her to come back next week when we are open." Bree said, before heading to the small office waiting room where she could see the shadow of someone outside the frosted glass front door.

Not wanting to scare the girl, Bree opened the door slowly then stepped out into the hall, shutting the door quietly behind her. The girl, looking closer to seventeen than eighteen if you ignored the heavily made-up face, was thin. Too thin.

The girl's eyes met Bree's and Bree knew the girl was about to make a run for it. Stepping in front of her, Bree tried to stop her, holding out her hands to the girl. "Wait. I just want to help you."

But Bree could see that the girl wasn't listening. As the girl rushed past her, pushing Bree over as she passed, Bree caught a glimpse of big brown eyes that were filled with terror.

Bree had never seen anything like the look on the girl's face, and on instinct she had pushed away from the wall and started after the girl when the office door opened and Knox rushed out, Lucretia following right behind him.

"What's going on?" he asked, grabbing a hold of Bree's arm to steady her.

"I'm not sure," Bree said, though her mind was flooded with a hundred scenarios, none of them good. "There was a girl, a teenager, but she ran as soon as I tried to talk to her."

Bree looked up into his eyes. "She's in danger, Knox. I don't know what kind, but she's afraid of something. Or someone."

"Maybe she came to the clinic for birth control or because she thinks she's pregnant and she's afraid her parents will find out. Let me see if I can find her," Knox said, then let go of her arm and headed down the hall toward the stairs at a jog.

While Lucretia went back to shut down the office, Bree waited for Knox to return. When she saw him coming back down the hall, alone, her hopes that he had caught up with the girl died.

"She had too much of a head start for you to catch her," Bree said when he walked up. "I've dealt with the teenagers at Legacy House and others while I was working in the hospital as a nurse. I haven't ever had one react that way. Not with that amount of fear."

She had been more likely to get attitude from her teenage patients, at least at first. It usually took a while before you would figure out that it was mostly fear of what their bodies were going through or how their lives were about to change that was responsible for those attitudes. But she'd never seen such a hopeless fear on anyone's face as she'd seen on that young girl's.

"Maybe she'll be back Tuesday, when the clinic is open again," Knox said, though he looked as worried as Bree. "There's nothing we can do about it now."

The phone alarm on Bree's watch went off, reminding her that she had to leave then or she'd be late for after-school pickup. Silencing it, she saw that Knox was studying her.

"You're not working a shift at the bar tonight, are you?" he asked. "You have to be back at Legacy Clinic tomorrow."

Was she imagining the censorship in his voice? Was he suggesting that she shouldn't be working at the bar when she had to be at the clinic the next day? "I only work at the bar when I have the next day off, but that's really not any of your business, is it?"

"I'm sorry. You're right. I just think working at the bar while you're doing your residency could be a problem. You need to be at your best, especially if you have a labor patient."

Bree chose to ignore the concern in his eyes. What right did this man have to judge her? She felt the anger at his words as it boiled out of her. She'd worked her butt off getting to where she was. She'd spent years juggling a child, school and a job. To suggest that she would do anything to jeopardize her career, or more importantly a patient, was insulting.

"You don't know anything about me, Knox." The heat in her face and the dangerous rate of her heart told her that she was about to go ballistic on the man. The anger drove her to take a step, then another. She was so close now that she would swear she could hear the beat of his heart. Or was that sound the beat of her own racing heart? Her breaths came faster as her eyes met his. Her hands came up to rest on his chest. They both stood there a minute while her anger warred with something else. Something more dangerous than her anger. For a second she couldn't remember where she was or why she was angry. All she knew was something changed in her, in him, when their eyes met. When his eyes dropped lower to rest on her lips, she felt herself sway toward him. Was he thinking about kissing her? She was surprised to find that she wanted him to. She wanted Knox to kiss her. It didn't make any sense, but she couldn't deny it. She was attracted to the last person she had these feelings for.

No. She couldn't do this. That was wrong. Nothing had changed between them. It was just something she had imagined. This was just a flood of hormones that had been brought on by her anger.

Her hands fell away from him. Her back stiffened. She forced her eyes away from him. She was too strong, too smart, to let a bunch of hormones take control of her like this.

Turning, she walked back into the clinic and grabbed her backpack, passing him where he still stood in the hallway. Refusing to look at him, she started toward the stairwell. She'd only gone a few feet before she heard him call after her.

"You're right. I don't know you, Bree," he called out behind her, "but I want to. I want to know everything about you."

Bree's feet faltered as her heart stuttered for a second. What did those words mean? And did she really want to know? She made her feet continue down the hall. While Knox might not know it, soon he would know more about her than he had ever dreamed possible. She just hoped that what was left between them when he did learn the truth about what she had done wasn't the nightmare she feared.

Knox knew that Bree was back to her old ways of avoiding him the next day. He'd hoped after the time they'd spent at the clinic, and after their talk at the bar, that things had changed between the two of them. Of course, it was probably his stupid confession that he wanted to get to know her better that had changed things. They'd just begun to get into a nice rhythm working together at the clinic, so why had he gone and ruined it? Maybe because it was the truth? Maybe because as they'd stood together in that hallway, with her hand pressed against his chest, all he could think about was wanting her to stay there, touching him. When she'd moved away from him, he'd felt the distance between them as acute as having a part of himself ripped away.

Bree Rogers not only fascinated him in a way no woman had ever done before, she also made him feel a longing he didn't know was possible. She was more pretty than beautiful, more sweet than sophisticated. In other words, nothing like the women he normally found himself attracted to. There was something special about her that he couldn't describe. And when she looked into his eyes it was as if she could see into his soul. He just wished he knew what it was she saw. Was it the boy he'd been who had never thought of others or of the consequences of what he did? Or was it the man he'd worked so hard to become? From the way she seemed to avoid him, he was afraid it was the former instead of the latter. Would he ever be able to put his past behind him?

"Do you have a moment, Knox?" Jack called out to him as Knox passed the senior Dr. Warner's office.

"Sure. I'm just headed over to the hospital to check on a postsurgical patient before I leave for the day. What's up?" Knox said, stepping into the older man's office.

"I know that you only have a few more weeks before your contract is up and Dr. Hennison returns. I just wanted to touch base with you and see what your plans were."

Knox took the seat in front of Jack's desk. "I've had some requests from some of the general practitioners up in the Smoky Mountains for me to return. I've been thinking of starting a type of travel practice where I can set up a home base in a central location, but still travel to some of the outlying areas where it's hard for people to get down to an office for a visit."

The two of them discussed the shortage of OB/GYN practices in the rural parts of the country for several minutes and what more the government could do to help encourage practitioners to move to those areas. Both of them agreed that a solution needed to be found for the women who didn't have access to the prenatal care they needed, due a lot to the cost of liability insurance.

"And what about Bree? How is she doing at the county clinic? I know she wasn't happy at first about the opportunity, but I thought the two of you would make a good team there. I hope you've been able to change her mind."

Knox was pretty sure that he'd destroyed the teamwork that they had been developing by admitting his interest in her, but he wasn't about to discuss that with Jack. And he knew she was mad at him over his questioning her about her need to work at the bar. He wasn't even sure if the practice was aware that Bree was working outside her commitment to them. But as he had been told, it wasn't his business. "She's doing well. The patients like her and she has a lot of empathy for their situation. Not everyone does."

"Well, that's good to hear. From everything I hear from Lori, she's going to make a good midwife," Jack said as his phone rang. Looking at the number, he shook his head. "It's my son. Always worrying I'm working too much."

"I have a mom for that. It's nice to know someone cares, isn't it?" Knox laughed, then stood and started out the door before Jack waved him to wait after telling his son to hold a moment.

"If you change your mind and decide to stay in town, let us know. We'd be happy to have you join the practice permanently," Jack said.

"It's a tempting offer, sir. Maybe one day I'll take you up on it. But for now, I think I'm needed in the mountains." He'd wondered if he'd get an offer from the practice and he hadn't been sure until that moment what he'd do if it came. Living close to his parents was tempting. His mother reminded him constantly that he wasn't getting any younger and needed to settle down. But just talking to Jack about the opportunity to make a difference in the rural communities of the mountains got him excited. That was where he was truly needed.

"I can't blame you for that. If I was twenty years younger, I think I'd join you. The mountains are beautiful this time of year and the work you're going to be doing will make a lot of difference for those communities," Jack said before returning to his call.

Knox stepped out the office door, only to find Bree standing in the middle of the hall.

"You're leaving?" she asked, her look intense and her tone demanding. "When?"

"I didn't know you cared," Knox teased, then stopped when he realized she was seriously upset. "I'm not leaving today. Jack just wanted to know my plans after I finish my contract here. What's wrong?"

Bree wasn't sure what was wrong. Knox's leaving was the answer to all her problems. If he wasn't there, the guilt she felt every time she looked at him would go away. Except, that wasn't true. She'd told herself that she was going to be honest with him. She was going to tell him about Ally. His leaving would complicate that in a lot of ways. The worst way being if he decided that he wanted to fight for custody of Ally and wanted to take her away with him, something that she hadn't considered until now. Her stomach protested at the thought, her insides doing a somersault. She couldn't face the possibility of Ally being taken from her.

But she couldn't explain any of this to Knox. Not yet. "I just need to know if I'll be working with you at the clinic for the next three weeks like we had planned."

"Like I said, I'm not leaving till my contract is over."

"Good," she said. She sounded like someone with only two functioning brain cells. "I mean, it's good that you'll be there to work in the clinic."

"Are you okay?" Knox asked, his eyes studying her too closely. "You look tired."

"Well, thank you for that. That's just what every woman wants to hear." After another night of tossing and turning, she hadn't been surprised to find the dark shadows under her eyes. She'd told herself that she wasn't sleeping because of her decision to tell Knox about Ally, but she'd awakened more than once from dreams about Knox that had her pushing the covers off her overheated body. She couldn't forget the way she'd felt when Knox had brushed his finger down her cheek. The way her body had responded when he'd just looked at her lips. If he'd kissed her at that moment, she would have gone up in flames.

"I'm just concerned about you. You're doing a lot between the clinic and working at the bar," said Knox, his eyes lingering on those shadows.

The concern in his voice just made her feel worse about her deception. Guilt was eating her up inside. She had to move forward with her plan to tell Knox about Ally. She had to ignore all other feelings she had for Knox and concentrate on the fact that he was her niece's father.

And the first thing she had to do was to introduce him to Ally. "Are you going to be at the cleanup day at Legacy House this weekend?"

"I'm planning on it," Knox said. "I think everyone that isn't on call is coming. It seems to be a big office project."

"That's good. It sounds like they'll need all the volunteers they can get," she said, then began walking backward, away from him. "I guess I'll see you there, then."

"Okay, it's a date," he said, giving her a smile that sent her libido into overdrive. Then the evil man winked at her before walking away, leaving Bree in shock as she stood and watched him go.

What had just happened? Was the man flirting with her now? He wasn't serious. He'd just been joking. Hadn't he? He didn't really think she'd been trying to get a date with him.

Slowly, she walked away, her mind filled with scenes of Knox Collins and his dangerously wicked smile.

CHAPTER FIVE

B<small>REE HELPED</small> A<small>LLY</small> pull the wagon they'd filled with small tree limbs the two of them had picked up from the backyard of Legacy House. She had told Ally that she wanted to introduce her to the doctor she worked with at the clinic, hoping to somehow smooth Knox and the little girl's introduction before she revealed to the two of them that they were father and daughter. Now the little girl asked every few minutes if "that doctor" was there yet. Bree was starting to think that she had been stood up, which was crazy. It wasn't a real date. Knox had just been teasing her. Still, she caught herself looking up from their work every time a new car drove into the driveway of the home.

They'd been working for almost an hour, when a dark blue truck stopped in front of the house and parked. Her breath caught when a jean-clad Knox climbed out. Dolly Parton's song about a man with a cowboy hat and painted-on jeans showing up to tempt her started playing in Bree's mind. Knox was every bit tempting as any man she had ever seen. He'd pulled his hair back into a tiny tail at the back of his head, giving him the look of a young rogue in one of her historical romances.

DEANNE ANDERS   81

"Aunt Bree, who's that guy? Is he your doctor?" Ally asked from beside her.

That question got her full attention. If someone had told her six months ago that she would be standing there, about to introduce Ally to the man who was her father, Bree would never have believed it. Knox's finding out about the little girl was a nightmare that she would have run from. But now, after getting to know him, she knew she was doing the right thing.

Not that she was going to tell either of them about their relationship yet. She had to go about that more cautiously. First, she wanted them to meet. She wanted Knox to see that Ally was a happy girl and that Bree was taking good care of her. Then she would tell him. After that, she'd see where they went. She thought that it would be best if Bree and Knox told Ally together, but that would all depend on how things went with Knox first. There was a probability that Knox would want to get a DNA test before he accepted that Ally was his. And while Bree had no doubt that Brittany had told the truth about Ally being his child, she couldn't blame him for wanting proof.

"He's not my doctor. He's the doctor I work with at the clinic downtown. The one I told you about. Do you want to meet him now?" Bree asked the little girl, who was studying Knox as he greeted one of the other volunteers. She watched as he opened the bed of his truck and began to remove bags of soil, throwing two of them over his shoulder before he headed their way.

"Sure," Ally said, then headed off to where some of

the other children were helping to pull the weeds out of a flower garden that ran the length of the front porch. It seemed Ally wasn't as impressed as Bree was by Knox's arrival.

She knew the moment he saw her, their eyes meeting and his lighting up as he gave her a grin before handing the bags of soil over to the man next to him and then returning back to the truck where he opened the back door. She watched as he reached into the backseat and came out with a small pot containing a beautiful royal blue orchid. Turning, he looked back at her, smiling as he headed toward her.

"I'm not usually late for my dates," he said, holding out the ceramic pot with the beautiful flower. "This is for you."

Bree looked at the potted plant, then back up at his smiling face. Had the man been serious when he'd called their meeting together today a date? Or was he still teasing her?

Guilt flooded through her system, as a nasty knot formed in her chest. What was she doing? She'd thought that getting to know Knox would be a good way to help her decide what to do about her niece, but the more she got to know him, the more she liked him. Now she thought of him as more than Ally's father, and more than just a work colleague. Now she was venturing into a place that could turn into a nightmare. The sooner she told Knox about Ally, the better for both of them. She just needed to give them time to get to know each other first. And she needed to build a relationship between her and Knox so that when she did approach him with the truth, he would be more open to listening to all the reasons she needed to remain as Ally's guardian.

Using that excuse, she reached out and took the plant, her hand brushing against Knox's, sending a tingle of awareness through her.

"What's that, Aunt Bree?" Ally asked from beside her, startling her. "Are you going to plant it in the flower beds?"

"Not this one," Bree said. "It's an orchid. We have to keep it inside and take good care of it."

"Well, hello," Knox said. "What's your name?"

Bree's heart expanded with something she refused to name at the kindness in Knox's eyes as he bent down to the little girl's level. Ally and Knox's first meeting would forever be a bittersweet memory that she hoped she would never feel the need to regret.

"I'm Ally. Are you Aunt Bree's doctor?" Ally asked, her face studying Knox's with a seriousness beyond her years.

"I'm one of the doctors your aunt works with," Knox said.

"Okay," Ally said, before turning to her aunt. "Is he the doctor you wanted me to meet?"

Knox stood and looked up at Bree, one eyebrow lifting as his lips turned up in a teasing smile. "Am I the doctor you wanted her to meet?"

Bree chose to ignore his teasing. "This is Dr. Collins, and yes, he's the doctor I've told you about. The one I work with at the clinic where the women come in for help."

"You didn't say he was pretty," Ally said, cutting her eyes to look over at Knox. "Don't you think he's pretty, Aunt Bree?"

Now the two of them were teasing her, surprising, since Bree had never known her niece to be teasing like this before. She was even more surprised to find that both Ally and Knox shared the same expression on their face. Both expectant. Both waiting to see what she was going to say next.

"Well, look at that," Bree said, adopting their playful manner, "I've never noticed before, Ally, but I think you might be right. He is kind of pretty."

Knox laughed and Ally giggled before running off to where one of the volunteers had started to help some of the kids spread the soil in the beds that they were preparing to plant flowers.

"I didn't know you had a niece," Knox said as they stood there together with Bree feeling awkward now that Ally wasn't there between them.

"I told you that you didn't know everything about me," Bree reminded him.

She could just blurt out the truth. Just spit out the words "Yes, I have a niece and she's your daughter," but she knew now was not the time. So instead, she changed the subject to something more comfortable. "I think we've finished cleaning up all of the backyard. Jared and Sky just hauled a truckload of limbs and leaves away. We just need to edge the sides of the driveway now."

Walking away, she grabbed a hoe one of the volunteers had brought out and began to work on one side of the driveway while Knox grabbed another tool and started on the other side. Together, they worked in silence. Soon, they were joined by some of the other staff members who had finished in the backyard. By the time they completed edging the drive, Jared and Sky were back and everyone began to fill the truck with the last of the yard trimmings. The junior Dr. Warner, Jared and his fiancée, Sky, left a few minutes later with the last truck full of leaves and limbs.

"I have to say I'm impressed with all the work that was done today," Knox said as he joined Bree as she headed to the backyard where the Legacy House mom, Maggie, had taken the volunteers' kids to play on the new equipment that had been donated for the children who sometimes came to stay with their moms.

"I'm impressed with Legacy House in general. Nashville is lucky to have a place like this. It's nice to see that not only the office staff, but the community comes together to help the women here, too." Legacy House was truly a community project. There had been hundreds of women over the years who had found a safe haven there until they could find a permanent home.

"The news is so filled with the negatives of society, but I think that most people want to help others if they can. I see it a lot when I'm working in the rural areas up in the mountains. Neighbors help their neighbors, but most of them are just as willing to help out a stranger." Knox stopped and took a seat at an old picnic table that was in need of a coat of paint, something that one of the volunteers had mentioned needing to tackle on their next cleanup day at the house.

"It sounds exciting to work up in the mountains, never knowing what you are going to encounter, but what is it really like?" She was stalling, not wanting to leave without him getting to spend more time with Ally, while at the same time she'd wanted to ask him about his work in the mountains since the first time she'd heard of his work there.

"It's not like the TV shows. I'm not riding a horse up the side of the mountain every day, though I did ride one once with a local doctor who had an elderly woman that he wanted me to see. Her son had taken her down to the local clinic one day and when the doctor had recommended that she have surgery for a prolapsed uterus, she'd left swearing never to come see him again. He thought maybe with a second opinion, she'd change her mind. Needless to say, she took one look at the two of us and slammed the door."

"Well, that had to be discouraging," Bree said. While she'd worked with some difficult patients, she had never had one refuse to at least listen to what she had to say.

"It happens. Besides, I got a nice horse ride through some of the most beautiful country in the world," Knox said.

"You got to ride a horse?" Ally asked.

Bree hadn't realized the girl had come up beside her and was listening to their conversation. As Ally was getting older, Bree knew she needed to be more aware of what she said when her niece was around.

"I did. He was a really nice horse, too," Knox said as Ally came to sit beside him.

"Can I ride him?" Ally asked, moving closer to Knox.

"You can't ride that horse. He's not mine. Besides, he lives a long way from here. But my parents have several horses at their ranch. If your parents are okay with it, maybe me and your aunt Bree can take you to see them."

"I don't have parents. I have Aunt Bree," Ally said before turning toward Bree. "Can we go see the horses?"

"We'll have to see," Bree said. Ally had always had a fascination with horses, even though she'd never been around one except for the ones at the county fair. And while she was happy that Knox and Ally had something to bond over now, taking Ally to Knox's parents' home? That came with complications she hadn't even considered. Not that she had anything against the couple. Bree had met them as a child. They both had been nothing but kind and encouraging to Bree and her sister when they were just starting out in their music career. But there was always the possibility that they would recognize Bree as one of the Rogers Sisters, wasn't there? Bree didn't think so. They'd only been twelve and she had changed a lot over those years. No longer was she the long-limbed, awkward little girl she'd been on those big, imposing stages. Still...

"That always means no," Ally said solemnly to Knox.

"I didn't say that..." Bree said, though the girl was right. Usually, it did mean the answer would be no.

"How about the three of us get something to eat together and we can talk about it then?" Knox asked, his eyes studying Bree.

Bree started to refuse; she could see that he had questions about Ally. He had to have figured out that she was raising Ally on her own. And the fact that she had never mentioned having a niece whom she was responsible for probably seemed strange, as if she had been hiding that fact. Of course, she had been. But explaining why might bring up questions she wasn't ready to answer. Not yet. She needed more time.

But still, this was an opportunity for them all to get to know each other. Wasn't that what she wanted? Didn't she need to see how Knox responded to having a child around?

"I think that would be great," she answered, surprising herself as much as her niece. "Where did you have in mind?"

Knox watched as Ally, Bree's niece, finished off her glass of chocolate milk. When the little girl looked up at him, a ring of chocolate circling her mouth, Knox thought she had to be the prettiest thing he had ever seen. With her aunt's strawberry blond hair and bright green eyes, Knox could have taken the child to be Bree's.

He couldn't understand why Bree had never mentioned that she was raising a child. Wasn't that something people just talked about? All the parents he knew couldn't talk about their children enough. He knew if he had a child, he'd probably be one of those parents, too.

Was it because Bree wasn't the child's mother? He didn't think so. He'd observed Bree in her interactions with their patients at the clinic. She had always been warm and caring. So why did it seem that she had been keeping Ally a secret until today? She had told him that he didn't know everything about her. He had known that. After all, they'd only known each other for a short period of time. Still, this was something he thought would have come out at some point in their conversations together. If not at work, at least when they'd met at the bar. It would have explained one of the reasons she was working there. Supporting herself and a child while in school would have been tough.

"Can I have some money for the jukebox?" Ally asked.

Before Bree could open her purse, Knox pulled out his wallet and handed her a five-dollar bill. "Do you want me to ask the lady at the register for change for the machine?"

"No, thank you. I can do it. I am eight years old, you know," the little girl said before turning and walking over to the counter where the waitress who had served their pizza stood.

"A little touchy about her age?" he asked Bree.

"Apparently, eight is the new twelve. At least, that seems to be what her and her friends think," Bree said, then sighed. "She's determined to grow up as fast as possible, while I just want the time to slow down so she can enjoy being a child for as long as possible."

"Weren't you like that? Eager to grow up? I know I was." It was just too bad that he had wasted so much of his life while he was growing up, making decisions that he wasn't old enough to make. He'd spent most of his teenage years rebelling against parents who had been too busy with their career to notice. He could only hope Ally wouldn't waste her childhood that way, because it was only later, when you grew up and looked back, that you realized what you had lost. But then Ally didn't have parents who were always gone on the road. It was easy to see the way that Bree interacted with her niece that the two of them were close.

"I guess I was," Bree said.

He watched as she stared into her half-empty glass. Was she thinking about mistakes she had made, just as he had? He knew so little about her, something that had never bothered him about other women. But whatever this fascination he had for Bree, it made him want to know everything. Even the tiny things. What was her favorite color? Her favorite movie? Did she even like movies? Maybe she preferred books. There was so much he wanted to know. "How did you end up with Ally? Did something happen to her parents?"

She looked at him for a moment, before her eyes dropped back to her drink. "Her mother, my sister, was injured in a car accident not long after Ally was born. She didn't survive. I've had Ally since she was a newborn."

"I'm sorry. That had to be hard." And explained so much, like the pain he'd seen in her eyes the night she'd sung at the bar. And that song. It had to be one she'd written about losing her sister. "So you've been raising her by yourself for eight years? It has to have been hard balancing school with raising a baby."

And Bree didn't have just school to worry about. She'd had to make a living, too. He knew she'd worked as a labor and delivery nurse; all midwives did at some point. Had she also been working at the bar then, too? "Where is her father? Doesn't he help you?"

"My sister..." Bree stopped midsentence and Knox could tell this wasn't something that was easy for her to talk about. He shouldn't have pushed her like he'd done.

"I'm sorry. It's none of my business. It's just that the thought of a man not supporting his daughter or the woman who had chosen to take care of his child, seems inexcusable to me."

"It's not like that," Bree said quickly. "It's complicated. My sister... Well, that's complicated, too."

"You don't have to tell me," Knox said. He didn't want Bree to feel like he was pressuring her to tell him all of her secrets, even though he wanted to know every single one.

"No, it's not that. I need to tell you this." Bree looked over to where Ally was picking out songs on the old-timey jukebox. "Ally's mother, my sister, she didn't feel that it would be a good thing for Ally's father to be involved in her daughter's life when she was born."

Knox didn't like the sound of that. "Was he abusive?"

"No, she never said that." Bree's voice sounded strange and he looked down to see her fingers had turned white as she gripped the table. "She just told me that he wouldn't want a baby and he would be a bad influence."

"So she never told him about the baby?" That didn't seem right to him. Didn't the man have a right to know? Even if he wasn't in a good place then, was it possible that knowing he had a child might have given him the encouragement to change?

"Look, I know it has to be hard talking about this. Your sister was young when you lost her, right?"

"She was my age," Bree said. "We were twins."

Twins. As an only child, he couldn't really appreciate what losing a sibling would be like, but it had to be hard. Losing a twin, someone you'd shared your whole life with, had to be even harder.

"Is it possible, then, that she might have changed her mind about Ally's father? Maybe they could have worked things out?" he said. "It just doesn't seem fair that he wasn't given that chance."

The small restaurant filled with music from a well-known pop star as Ally rushed back over to them, cutting their conversation off.

Knox could see that Bree's niece was a happy, well-adjusted child, even after what had to be a rough start to her young life. He had no doubt it was because Ally had been lucky enough to have someone like Bree to take care of her.

And though it seemed wrong that Bree's sister hadn't told Ally's father about the pregnancy, it wasn't any of his business. It sounded as if the mother had been looking out for her child. What more could a parent do?

"Are you two talking about horses again?" Ally asked as she flung herself into the seat beside her aunt.

"No, we weren't. But if the invitation is still open, I think it would be a great idea for you to go see his parents' horses."

Knox was surprised by Bree's about-face on his invitation, but he wasn't about to lose the chance to spend more time with the two of them, as he was discovering that Ally was almost as enchanting as her aunt. "Are the two of you by any chance free tomorrow?"

That night, as Bree climbed into bed, she looked over to where a picture of her sister sat on her nightstand. Was she doing the right thing? Did she have a choice? She couldn't continue living with the knowledge of how her promise to her sister had affected Knox and Ally.

She picked up the picture of Brittany and a wave of grief hit her. How many nights had she cried herself to sleep while she was holding this picture? How long was she going to put herself through this? It was time to do the right thing for both Ally and Knox. And it was time to let go of the grief and guilt that she'd felt ever since Brittany had died.

She would always love and miss her sister. And even though they'd grown apart, Bree knew that Brittany had still loved her. Her sister wouldn't want her to keep going through this pain, night after night.

"I love you, Brittany," she said before setting the picture down, "and I'm sorry I have to break my promise to you, but I can't keep doing this. Ally deserves to know her father and Knox deserves to know his daughter."

Bree wiped away the tears from her eyes and took a

shaky breath. "I will never forget you. You will always be my sister. But from now on, I'm going to concentrate on the good times we had, instead of what we lost. Because I deserve to be happy, too."

CHAPTER SIX

BY THE TIME Bree had gotten Ally ready for their trip to Knox's parents' ranch, her mind had come up with a dozen ways that what she was about to do could go wrong. What if Knox was so angry at her that he went to Dr. Warner and had her thrown out of the practice? What if his parents called one of their lawyers and had Ally taken away from her?

The doorbell sounded. It was too late to cancel now. Ally checked the door monitor as she'd been taught before skipping away to let Knox in. Bree rubbed her damp hands down her jeans. She had to make herself relax. She was doing the right thing.

Now that she'd cracked open a can of worms, she knew that it could be thrown wide open for the whole world to see by the end of that day. Scared of what might follow, she wanted to take her niece and hide in her closet. But she'd made her peace with her decision the night before. It was time for her to face Knox and tell him the truth.

Squaring her shoulders, she pasted a smile on her face as Knox walked inside, Ally beside him with her mouth going a hundred miles an hour.

"Sorry, she's been like this ever since she got up this morning," Bree said. "Ally, run and get your backpack."

As the girl ran off, twin pigtails flying behind her, Knox laughed. "She has a lot more energy than me at this time of the day."

"Me, too. Would you like a cup of coffee?" Bree asked, turning away from him and heading to the kitchen. She was finding it hard to look Knox in the eyes, something that didn't bode well for the rest of the day. She had to calm down. Trying to anticipate what his reaction to learning about Ally would be was too much. She just needed to take this one step at a time. The first thing to do was to get it over with, but there was no chance at that while Ally could interrupt them at any moment.

Right then, the little girl flew into the room. With eyes bright with excitement, she reminded Bree so much of Brittany right before she performed. It was pure, innocent joy on Ally's face, and Bree was so afraid she was about to destroy all of that if she didn't handle this right.

"Can we go now?" Ally begged, pulling on the leg of Knox's jeans.

"It looks like I'll need that coffee to go," Knox said, looking down at Bree's little girl, his own face just as happy-looking as the child's, before he looked back up at her.

With that one look, Bree's stomach unknotted and her body relaxed. Knox didn't even know that Ally was his child, yet Bree could see how much he enjoyed being around her. No matter how Knox took the news, as long as he loved Ally, it would be okay. Even though she knew that Bree and Knox's relationship would never be the same, it would all be worth it for Ally and Knox to have the life they deserved.

"Are we almost there?" Ally asked as Knox turned his truck down a small lane that led to his parents' ranch. She'd been asking the same question for the past thirty minutes, her excitement increasing with each mile.

"Almost. Keep looking over on your right and you might see a horse or two in the field," Knox said, then looked over at Bree. "I'm afraid of what she might do when she finally sees one of the horses."

"We had a talk about behaving around the horses this morning when she got up, but it would probably be a good idea for you to tell her, too." Bree wasn't really worried about Ally's safety. She knew that Knox wouldn't let her niece around any of the horses that were dangerous.

"I will. And I talked to the ranch manager, Rodney, about bringing the two of you out today. He was going to pick out a pony for Ally. I wouldn't take a chance with either of your safety."

"I know that," Bree said, and knew there was truth in his words. No matter what her sister had thought of Knox when he was younger, he wouldn't do anything to hurt Ally. Not intentionally at least.

Ally let out a squeal and began hopping up and down in her seat. "I see one, I see one."

Bree looked over to where her niece was pointing and saw a pretty brown-and-white horse standing in the field.

A few minutes later, they came to a halt in front of a

large red metal barn. Before Bree could get out of the car, Ally had freed herself from her seat and was running toward it.

"Whoa, there," Knox said, catching up to Ally and stopping her, before taking a knee in front of her. "I know your aunt Bree told you that you needed to be careful around the horses. Running up to them is not being careful. You could spook one of them and they could hurt you or themselves."

"I don't want to hurt the horses," Ally said as her chin began to tremble, and big fat tears rolled down her cheeks.

Knox looked up at Bree with something akin to horror in his face. "I didn't mean to make her cry."

The man could handle all kinds of emergency situations in the operating room, but one little girl's tears scared him like this?

"It's okay, Ally. We know you don't want to hurt the horses. Knox just wants to make sure you are safe. And we did discuss no running around the horses this morning, didn't we?" Bree asked her niece.

"Yes, ma'am," Ally said, using her shirtsleeve to wipe at her face before turning toward Knox. "I'm sorry, Dr. Knox. I won't run and scare the horses. I promise."

"That's okay," Knox said, standing and holding out a hand to Ally. "Let's go see some of my parents' horses. And then I have a surprise for you."

When Ally took Knox's hand, then looked up at him with eyes full of trust, Bree's heart was filled with so much love that she felt as if it might burst out from her chest. She realized then that it wasn't just Ally she was feeling that love for, it was also for the man who held her niece's hand. How had her feelings for him changed so much, so fast? It was as if everything in the universe had thrown them together at just the perfect time.

"You coming?" Knox asked, looking back at her, then stopping as he studied her face. Did he see how much his simple act of taking her niece's hand in his had affected her? Could he see how much her own reaction to him was changing? Did he feel this way, too?

Not that it mattered. She couldn't make this about her and Knox. She had to remember that her focus had to be on Ally and Knox's relationship, not the way that her heart sped up every time he looked at her, just like the way he was looking at her now.

"Come on," he said, holding out his other hand to her. Was it wrong for her to wish everything could be different between them? That she could take what he offered her, the friendship and maybe more, without knowing that soon he might hate her for all the years of his daughter's life that she stole from him?

Unable to help herself, she reached out and took his hand. Its warmth calmed her. And for the next half hour she held on to it, wishing she would never have to let it go as he took them through the horse stables, pointing out one horse after another. Ally's excitement grew with each new horse they saw, but she stayed close to them as Knox had instructed her, while staff members went about their work hauling hay and cleaning the stalls.

"And this is where we keep my mother's ponies," Knox said when they got to the end of the stalls.

"Isn't your mom too big to ride a pony?" Ally asked as they stopped by an older man who was saddling up a small black pony.

"Mrs. Collins keeps the ponies around so that when little girls like you come over, you will be able to ride them," the man said, then removed his hat, exposing a bald head that was sporting a fresh sunburn, as he held out a hand for Bree to shake. "I'm Rodney, ma'am."

Letting go of Knox's hand, she took the man's hand, noting its rough callouses that reminded her of her father's. "It's nice to meet you, Rodney. I'm Bree. And this is Ally."

"It's nice to meet you both. This here is Sammy. He's a nice little pony that likes little girls. Do you want to pet him, Ally?"

With a nod from Bree, Ally approached the pony slowly, before placing her hand on the top of its head like Rodney showed her.

"I think it's love at first sight," she whispered to Knox when he stepped closer.

"I think so, too," he said. But when she looked up at him, she noticed that it was she he was looking at, instead of her niece. Her hand shook when his hand reached down for hers again. She let him take it. Why couldn't she enjoy a few moments before everything came crashing down around her?

They stood and watched Ally get her first lesson on how to saddle the pony before Rodney helped her up onto the pony's back and led her out of the barn and into an adjoining paddock.

"There you are." A loud feminine voice came from behind them. Turning, Bree saw Gail Collins approaching. The years since Bree had seen her had been good to her. Though there was a little gray in the woman's long dark blond hair, her face carried very few wrinkles. Dressed in jeans and sporting a rhinestone belt buckle, she still looked like the Country Music Queen she'd been all those years ago when Bree had met her.

"Bree, this is my mom," Knox said as the beautiful woman stretched up on her toes and planted a noisy kiss on his cheek. Instead of shrugging off her attention, Knox wrapped his free arm around her. "Mom, this is Bree Rogers. She's the midwife who has been working with me at the county clinic."

"It's nice to meet you, Bree," Knox's mother said before stepping back and studying Bree. "Have we met before?"

Bree knew that this time would come. She was bound to meet Knox's mother someday. Yet, she still hadn't decided on how to handle it. With the exception of telling Knox about Ally, she had always stuck to the truth. It seemed best to do that now. "Yes, ma'am, but I doubt you'd remember me. I was only twelve years old at the time. My sister and I used to perform when we were kids. We were known as the Rogers Sisters."

"I remember now. The two of you were twins, not identical, though you did look similar."

"It was the hair and eyes," Bree said, shooting a look

over at Knox, waiting for him to put the two things together. Hadn't Brittany told him about her childhood
career?

"And you're a midwife now?" the woman said, still
studying her.

"Yes, ma'am. I'm just finishing up my residency now."

"And your sister?" Knox's mother asked. "Did she
leave the business, too?"

"Mom, Bree's sister was killed right after her daughter, Bree's niece, was born," Knox said, cutting into what
was starting to feel like an inquisition. "That's the little girl, Ally, that I told you I was bringing to see the
horses. We were just about to walk outside so we could
watch Rodney work with Ally. He has her on Sammy."

"I'm so sorry, Bree. Please excuse me from asking
so many questions. It's just so rare for Knox to bring
a woman out here to meet us. I just want to know all
about you. And it's so interesting that we met when you
were a child."

Bree looked over at Knox and caught him rolling his
eyes at his mother's statement. His mother changed the
subject to ponies and horses, then circled back to her
hopes that someday she would have grandchildren to
teach to ride all the horses she'd collected. Bree wanted
to laugh at the woman's not so subtle hints that Knox
needed to get busy in the baby-making department.

But once they reached the paddock, the woman
stopped talking and just stared where Ally sat on the
pony, listening carefully to every word Rodney said.
Never had Bree seen her niece look so serious.

"She's beautiful, Bree," Knox's mother said from behind her. "And a natural in the saddle. Look how perfectly she's seated. She'll make a great rider."

Bree didn't know what to say to that, so she just stood there, still holding Knox's hand, and watched as her niece took one more step away from her into a life that Bree would never be able to give her.

Fifteen minutes later, she could see that Ally was getting tired. Fortunately, Gail Collins could see it, too. "Let me go get her back to the stable."

When Bree started to follow her, Knox pulled her aside. "I'm sorry if my mother upset you with her questions about your sister. She didn't mean to."

"I know that. She had no way of knowing," Bree said, wanting to say so much more. She suddenly needed to get all of this off her chest, once and for all. Both Knox's and his mother's kindness was just too much. She didn't deserve any of it.

She pulled her hand from his, feeling the loss immediately. Then she wrapped her arms around herself, unexpectedly cold while in the warmth of the summer sun.

"I need to talk to you. Privately." The words sounded more ominous than she'd meant them to and the whole mood of the day changed as Knox looked at her, his eyes worried.

"I asked my mother to have a picnic fixed for the two of us. I thought I could show you some of the ranch and I know my mom would love to spend time with Ally. That is, if you would like that," Knox said as they walked back into the stable where they were greeted by a smiling Ally and Knox's mother.

"Ms. Gail says I can come to her house and see her horse collection," Ally said. "They aren't real horses, but she says some of them have pink and purple ribbons I can braid in their hair."

"That sounds like a lot of fun. But you have to be careful and not break them," Bree told her niece.

"I'll run in and get the food. Then we can go down to the pond," Knox said. "Or you can come up to the house with me if you would like."

Bree followed him out of the barn where she could see the two-story house that stood to the north. It was a beautiful house. And just one more thing to remind her that Knox and his parents could give Ally so much more than she could.

Around her, the fields of grass swayed with the summer breeze. Even with the voices of the workers in the stables, there was a calming quietness there that she needed. "No, I'll wait here."

She strode over to a fencerow and placed one boot-clad foot on the first fence post she came to, welcoming this short period of time she had alone with her thoughts. She was going to do this. She had no other choice. Even without seeing her niece walk off, hand in hand with the grandmother she had never known, Bree knew coming clean with Knox about Ally had to be done now. Her and Ally's time alone together was up.

It was only a few minutes before she heard the sound of a small motor headed her way. She turned to see Knox driving an all-terrain cart toward her, a basket sitting beside him.

"Climb in," Knox said when he stopped and moved the basket to the back floorboard.

Bree took the seat beside him, buckling herself in before Knox started down the drive. He then took a right turn down a worn path through an open field running beside another paddock, this one larger with a taller fence.

She grabbed a handle above her as they drove over the rocky path at a speed that at first scared her, then became thrilling. By the time they had arrived by a large pond, they both were laughing.

For a moment, Bree forgot that she was about to spill a secret that would change all their lives. When Knox bent his head toward hers, she knew she should stop him, but she couldn't find the strength to turn her head away. As his lips brushed against hers in a gentle kiss, she closed her eyes and made a wish for her and Knox to someday get a second chance. When she opened her eyes, she found Knox's face still close to hers. Her hand cupped his cheek, the day's stubble rough against her skin.

"Something's bothering you, Bree. Is it those questions from my mom? She didn't mean to bring up bad memories," Knox said, his eyes watching her with an intensity she'd never experienced. It wasn't the first time she'd seen him like this. It was as if he was memorizing everything about her in that moment. As if he wanted to sink into her soul and know all her secrets.

And now he was about to learn more than he could ever have imagined.

"It's not that, not really. I've decided that instead of thinking about those bad memories, I need to concentrate on the good ones. Over the years, I've let the loss of my sister define our relationship, and I shouldn't have. Does that make sense?" She didn't know why she was telling him this, but it seemed important that he understand that she was making changes in her life. Looking at things differently. Just like she was looking at him differently now.

"It makes a lot of sense. Everybody handles the grieving process in different ways and in different time frames. But if that isn't what's bothering you, what is it?"

"Can we have just a few more minutes before I tell you?"

"Of course we can," Knox said, moving away from her and reaching over for the basket. When she joined him, he took her hand and led her down to where a weather-beaten wood pier had been built across part of the pond. When they got to the end of the pier, he put the basket down, then sat down beside it. Hanging his feet over the end of the pier, he offered Bree a hand and she took a seat beside him before looking out at the lake with its mirror-smooth surface. It was the calm before the storm.

Opening the basket, Knox pulled out sandwiches and drinks, laying them between them, along with some fruit. Her stomach was queasy, but she forced herself to unwrap a sandwich and take a bite. She wasn't sure if her stomach was reacting to her nerves about what she was about to do or if it was because of the kiss they'd just shared.

They ate in silence as they both looked out across the water. A fish hit the top of the water startling Bree and causing her to jump and let out a nervous laugh. The hollowness of it seemed to echo across the lake.

"I don't know where to start. I know I should start at the beginning, but I can't say I even know where this all began. Maybe you can help me with that."

"I'd be glad to help you if I can," Knox said, turning toward her, laying his sandwich down. "Maybe if you tell me what's wrong, the two of us can fix it."

Bree looked at him sitting there beside her. He was so calm. So reassuring. It was hard to believe he was the same man that her sister had been so adamant that he wouldn't be good for her child.

Bree had made such a big mistake all those years ago, not giving him a chance to prove that he would be a good father.

"I'm going to tell you everything I know, and then maybe you can help fill in some of the blanks for me. You see, before my sister died, I hadn't heard from her in over eighteen months even though we lived in the same city."

"I'm sorry to hear that. Families can be so complicated," Knox said. "But I don't know where I come in."

"I know you don't. And that's my fault, not yours. I should have told you this months ago." She looked away from him then, seeking the calm she'd felt from their surroundings earlier, but it didn't come. Maybe she didn't deserve it. Maybe she deserved all the sleepless nights, and guilty nerves she'd suffered for the past few weeks.

"No. That's not right. I should have told you this years ago. But I didn't know you then. And I'd made a promise I didn't think I could break."

When Knox started to interrupt her, she rested a hand on his chest. "Do you even remember my sister?"

Knox stared at Bree. She was talking in circles, making it impossible to figure out what it was that she was trying to tell him. Her sister? Why would he remember her sister?

"She had dyed her hair, it was more red than blond the last time I saw her, but she would still have had my eyes. She still went by her first name, Brittany. But she had changed her last name to Moore. She didn't want people to remember her from our childhood performance."

The name was vaguely familiar, but why? Then it hit him. "She was working at one of the recording studios as a backup singer. I remember her. She hung out with some of the music crowd I knew. I didn't know her that well…" A memory surfaced then. Red hair. Beautifully haunting green eyes. It was the night he and Thad had been out partying. She had been with the group of his parents' band members whom Knox had stayed back with when Thad had left the bar. As it always did, thoughts of Thad brought back all his old grief and guilt. He talked a good talk with Bree about grieving, but he was still struggling himself with the loss of his friend.

And the girl? He remembered meeting her at the bar that night, and then the two of them sharing a car ride. Later, at his place, they had shared more. Was that what this was all about? Did Bree know that her sister had spent the night with him? "She went by Britt," he said. "I guess like the way you go by Bree, instead of Brianna."

"She did go by Britt, sometimes. It was usually only with people she was close to, though," Bree said, her eyes looking at him expectantly, like he had the answer to a question he didn't know.

Or was she just waiting for him to admit that he had slept with her sister? His life then had been so different. He'd lived it one day at a time, never thinking about the consequences. That is, until the night Thad was killed.

"I don't know what your sister told you, but back then, when I met your sister, I wasn't the same person I am now. I was young and reckless. There are a lot of things I wish I had done differently then. I'm sorry if the night I spent with your sister upsets you. It's not something I'm proud of." Revisiting that night was a nightmare. He and Thad had started partying early that day and hadn't had the good sense to stop. If it hadn't been for who his parents were, he was sure the bars would have thrown them out on the streets.

But then, if his parents hadn't been who they were, he might not have acted out the way he had. It hadn't been until he reached rock bottom that he and his parents had realized how unhealthy their relationship had become. Thank goodness they'd been able to work things out then, before there was any more damage to their relationship.

But that night had been before he'd come to his senses. He could barely remember the girl he now knew as

Bree's sister, offering to get him home. It wasn't until that morning when he'd received the call that Thad was in the hospital with little hope of surviving, that Knox had finally sobered up. He'd left Bree's sister in his bed without an explanation and hadn't returned until the next night. He was ashamed to say that he hadn't given Brittany another thought, until now.

It was like all his sins were coming back to revisit him when he looked over at Bree. How did he tell her that he'd known her sister, but all she'd meant to him was one night of drunken pleasure?

"I don't know what your sister told you about me. I can tell you that I'm not the man I was then and I'm ashamed of the way I acted that night. I wish I could say that there weren't any more women like her, one-night stands with women I barely knew, but I can't. I can use my youth as an excuse, but I don't want to make excuses. I learned the hard way that you have to take responsibility for your actions and face the consequences. I did that many years ago, but sometimes those consequences last for years."

"I don't understand. Are you saying that Brittany was just a one-night stand? Because that isn't how she acted. She acted like the two of you had been together and it had ended badly. I took it to mean that the two of you were involved."

Knox looked over at Bree. Her face was pale, her pupils almost pinpoint. She looked as if she was in shock as she stared at him. Gone was the warmth he was used to seeing in her eyes. She looked like she'd seen a ghost.

The ghost of her sister? Because right then he felt like Brittany was standing there between the two of them.

How did he fix this without making it look like he was calling her sister a liar? Had he said something that would have made Brittany think that there was more between the two of them? How could that even be possible when he'd never seen her again?

After Thad's death, he'd applied himself to finishing his exams. And when the guilt and depression from Thad's death had threatened to send him back into his bad ways, he'd checked himself into a rehab. He'd cut all ties then, only taking calls from his parents until he'd found the help he needed to get his life onto a path he was proud of.

"I'm sorry, Bree. I don't want to hurt you or suggest that Brittany wasn't truthful, but the only thing that me and Brittany shared was one night together. That was all."

Knox started to gather the leftover meal wrappers. This was not the way he had planned for the two of them to end the day. When Bree's hand closed over his as he reached for the last of their mostly uneaten meal, he looked up at her, expecting to see anger, disgust, or the coolness she'd treated him to the first months they'd worked together.

But there was none of those things. Instead, there was sorrow and regret. "But that wasn't all you shared, Knox. The two of you shared Ally."

CHAPTER SEVEN

THERE WAS NO laughing on their ride back to the ranch house, as Knox shot off question after question at her. Bree couldn't blame him for the anger she could see brewing in his eyes.

"How is that possible?" he asked, then shook his head when she didn't answer. He was an OB/GYN; he knew how pregnancy happened as well as she did.

"Okay, let's say I am Ally's father. Why wouldn't Brittany have told me?" he asked, then answered the question himself before she could answer. "She would have found out about the pregnancy when I was away in rehab. I didn't have my phone with me. Only my parents knew how to contact me. But after? When Ally was born? I would have been out then. She should have called then."

"I told you I had a lot of blanks I needed you to fill in. I only talked to her the once in eighteen months. She hadn't told me anything about the pregnancy. I don't have any proof of this, but I've always thought that she might have been considering giving up Ally. Maybe that's why she didn't tell either of us? Maybe it wasn't until Ally was born that she decided to keep her. We've both seen that happen before."

Knox swerved around a rock in the middle of the path, causing Bree to grip the over-the-head handle even tighter.

"Maybe we should stop." He'd been driving full throttle since he'd insisted that they get back to the ranch as soon as possible. He was upset. Shocked. But so was she.

Learning that her assumption that Brittany and Knox had been involved in a relationship was wrong changed everything. What if Ally wasn't even Knox's child? She hadn't been able to say those words out loud, but he had to be thinking them, too.

Was it possible? Could it be that Brittany had made that part of her story up, too? The answer to that question tore Bree in two. On one hand, if Knox wasn't Ally's father, Bree could let go of the guilt she'd felt at assuming that he wasn't fit to be. And if Knox wasn't Ally's father, she wouldn't have to worry about losing Ally. On the other hand, that would mean that there was another man out there who could someday challenge Bree for her niece. A man who wouldn't be as kind and caring as Knox. A man who might not be good for her niece.

Being honest with herself, Bree knew that Ally having Knox for a father would be good for her. And she had to admit that it would be best if her niece's paternity was settled sooner instead of later.

Knox stopped the cart, but he didn't look at her. "We need a plan. We can't tell my mother this. And I know we can both agree that we can't tell Ally until we know for sure that I'm her father. There's places in Nashville that can run a paternity test in a day. We need to get that done first." He turned his head to her, his eyes somber now. "And then we need to have a long talk, no matter what the results."

The rest of their time at the ranch seemed to fly by as Knox did everything but rush them out to his truck. She started to stop him and ask if he thought she was going to just blurt out the news that Ally was his child to his mother or if he just couldn't stand to be around her anymore, but she was afraid to hear his answer.

He was angry and confused. She got that. She was, too. Just like him, she wanted to know the truth about her niece.

And she was also afraid. Only this time it wasn't the fear that she'd spoken to Lucretia about, the fear of losing Ally. This was a new fear. Something she was ashamed to admit because it was so selfish of her. What right did she have to fear that what she and Knox had begun to feel for each other had been destroyed when he was now faced with the fact that he had trusted her and she had betrayed him by not sharing Brittany's secret with him?

By the time Knox dropped her and Ally off at their home, Bree had come to accept that there was little hope that Knox would forgive her, even if Ally wasn't his child. There had to be trust in any relationship, especially one as new as theirs. She could try to make excuses for her actions all day long, but the man who'd driven them home without even looking at her once was not going to listen to them. And she couldn't blame him.

* * *

The new week started off with a stop by a local lab where Bree could pick up a DNA paternity test. She had asked Knox to let her explain to Ally, but Bree still didn't know how to do that. While Bree believed in being truthful, she didn't think her niece was old enough to understand DNA or what it was used for. She'd finally decided in the middle of the night that it was best, for now, to just tell Ally it was a test she needed.

The rest of the day had gone by quickly with Bree and Lori attending two deliveries, one of which Bree was primary. The good thing about being busy was that it didn't give her a lot of time to think about her own problems. She'd only seen Knox once in the clinic hallway, but they'd both been too busy to stop and talk.

It wasn't until the next day, after she'd carefully swabbed Ally's cheek then dropped her off at school, that Bree had time to worry about the outcome of the paternity test. When she walked into the county clinic, she went straight to the back office and took the safely packaged test from her backpack. Knowing she could trust Lucretia not to snoop, she put the test in a paper bag and added a note to let Knox know it was for him.

A few minutes later, Knox stopped by Lucretia's desk where she and Bree were discussing supply list changes. After nodding his head toward the exam rooms, Bree followed him. He handed her the paper bag that contained the test, and she slipped it into her pocket. She couldn't help but smile at the way they were treating this.

"I feel like I should have a hat and fake mustache.

Maybe a trench coat, too," Bree said, hoping that she could lighten up the situation.

"I'd like to see you in a trench coat," Knox said, surprising Bree with the teasing comeback before turning serious again. "How did it go with Ally? She ask anything about the test?"

"Not at all. I admit I was surprised. I wasn't sure what I was going to say if she asked me what the test was for. I've always been honest with her about everything, but sometimes you can't tell someone everything you want to. Sometimes things are more complicated than the simple truth."

"If you are talking about your not telling me about Ally, I know there were reasons you didn't tell me. You made a promise to your sister, and then she passed away. But I don't understand how, after you met me, after you saw that I wasn't a bad person, you didn't tell me then. Why, Bree? Didn't you think I deserved to know if Ally was my child?"

How could she make him understand the weight of her sister's secret that she had carried for years? How could she expect him to forgive her for not telling him? "It was the last thing I told her, Knox. The last thing I said to my sister. I promised her that I wouldn't tell anyone about who was Ally's father."

She walked the length of the small exam room, then turned and started back to him. "Until this weekend I had never broken that promise. I had held my sister's secret deep inside and never dreamed of telling anyone the truth about Ally. Until I met you. And though I'm not proud of it, if you had been the type of man Brittany had accused you of being, I wouldn't have told you then. The only person I had ever considered telling Brittany's secret to was Ally when she got old enough to make her own decisions about the information her mother had given me."

"So, what? When she was eighteen or nineteen, she'd have suddenly showed up on my doorstep? Would that have been fair to either of us?" Knox asked, coming to stand in the path where she had been pacing the floor.

"Nothing about this situation is fair to any of us," Bree said, stopping in front of him. "It wasn't fair that Brittany was killed in an accident before she had the chance to raise her child. Who knows? Maybe once she had Ally at home, she would have changed her mind. But we'll never know that, will we?"

"You're right," Knox said, running his hands through his hair where it had fallen down in front of his face. "This hasn't been fair for anyone."

Bree heard a door shut and then Lucretia talking to someone who would be their first patient of the day. Holding the brown paper bag up in front of her, she nodded at Knox. "But at least with this we will have the truth."

Because until they found out if Knox was really Ally's father, there was no way for them to move forward.

Bree rushed back to put the test in her backpack before following Knox to the front of the office to greet their patient. By the time Bree got there, other patients had begun to file into the waiting room. The little office was soon full again, as it had been every day that Bree had been there. While Bree was glad to be busy, she hated that there were so many women who couldn't afford to get care. They provided what they could, but it wasn't the same.

For her last appointment of the day, Lucretia brought back a woman in her midthirties, along with an elderly woman whose eyes darted around the room, taking everything in. "This is Leah and her grandmother."

"It's nice to meet you both. What brings you to the clinic today?" Bree asked, still watching the older woman who was acting uneasy.

"My grandmother, Camila, she doesn't speak English. She has a knot, a lump, in her breast. I don't know where to take her to get this looked at. My sister says she needs a mammogram, but where do we get this?" The younger woman looked at Bree with worried eyes and Bree instantly understood her concerns.

Bree had lost her own mother to breast cancer. If her mother had gone to get her yearly exam, the cancer would have been caught earlier and her mother might still be alive today. "If it's okay with you and your grandmother, I'd like to give her an exam. That way we can make sure there isn't any other issue that we need to investigate. Then I'll get a mammogram scheduled."

After giving the woman a thorough exam, Bree left them in the exam room while she went to find Lucretia. She knew that there were programs run by the local hospitals to help women get their yearly mammogram, but she wasn't sure where the information was.

"I'm glad you're here," Lucretia said when Bree stepped into the reception office. "There's someone outside the office pacing back and forth. I think it's that young girl. The teenager from last week."

Bree stepped into the waiting room and looked out the door. She could see the shadow of someone outside the frosted door, standing against the back wall of the hallway. It was possible that it was someone waiting for a patient to finish, maybe another grandchild of Camila's, but Bree didn't think so. She'd waited all day for the frightened girl who had run away to come back. Bree was pretty sure that she had.

Bree went over to the reception window. She didn't want to let the girl get away before she could talk to her, but she also didn't want Leah or Camila to think she had forgotten about them. "Can you find the information for the free mammogram programs at the hospital and make an appointment for the patient in my exam room? Her granddaughter has all her contact information. It could be benign, but there is definitely a large mass in her right breast that needs to be seen to immediately. I'm going to ask Knox to recommend a surgeon who will work with them on finances once we get the results of the mammogram back."

"I can do that," Lucretia said. "What are you going to do?"

"I'm going to see if it's our returning patient. If it is, I'm not going to let her get away this time." Bree started toward the door. "Don't let anyone else out this door until I tell you to."

"Maybe we should call the police? What if she's dangerous? She pushed you over last time she was here," Lucretia said, leaning over the reception window.

"She's not dangerous. She was just scared."

"Wait," Lucretia said, holding out a pack of peanut butter crackers, "take these."

"You're the best," Bree told Lucretia, taking the crackers and heading back to the door. Maybe if she couldn't talk the girl into coming inside, she could bribe her.

She opened the door and stepped into the hallway, leaving the door open for a second while she waited to see what the girl's reaction was. Bree had denied to Lucretia that the girl was dangerous, but what did she really know about her? Fear made people do things that they normally wouldn't do. It had certainly caused Bree to make some bad decisions.

When the girl didn't run, Bree closed the door behind her, then held out the crackers. Once again, Bree noted the fear in the girl's eyes. "We thought you might like these."

The girl stared at the simple package of crackers like it was steak and lobster before looking at Bree with suspicion. "It's okay. They're for you."

"What do I have to do for them?" the girl asked, her young face transforming from that of a child's to a hardened adult in seconds. Bree had no doubt now that this girl was being abused in some way.

"You don't have to do anything," Bree said, coming to stand against the wall across from the girl. She wanted to take the girl into her arms and promise her she'd keep her safe, but that would only frighten the girl more. "You don't even have to talk to me if you don't want to."

When the girl reached for the crackers, Bree leaned forward toward her, then moved back away from her again. She wanted to cry when she saw the girl rip open the package of crackers and stuff the first one into her mouth. She wanted to go inside the office and get more for the girl to eat, but she was still afraid the girl would bolt on her.

When the girl finished the crackers and didn't run, Bree decided to take a chance. At some point someone was going to have to come out the office door and she didn't know how the girl would react. "Do you want something to drink? We have all kinds of bottled drinks inside. I can get you one if you don't want to come inside."

The girl's head shot up at the mention of a drink, her eyes coming to rest on the office door. Bree could tell that she wanted to go inside. The girl had come there for help. Bree just had to find a way to make her feel safe. "My name is Bree. I just started here as a midwife in training, but I can tell you that this is a safe place. No one is going to make you do anything you don't want to do here. But if you need help, you've come to the right place. We help people with all kinds of problems and we keep everything confidential. It's what we do."

"I'm Christine," the girl said, barely above a whisper, her voice sounding raw as if she hadn't used it in a while.

"Well, Christine, do you want to come inside with me? I don't mind talking in the hallway, but our office would be more private." When the girl didn't move, Bree continued. "I know you're scared. That's okay. I've been scared, too. Sometimes trusting someone is the scariest thing of all."

The girl pushed away from the wall, then stood staring at Bree. They stood there looking at each other for almost a minute, before big fat tears began to run down the girl's face and her body began to shake. "My name isn't Christine. That's the name the people who took me told me to use. My real name is Megan. Megan Johnson, and all I want is to go home. Can you help me?"

Knox walked out of an exam room where he had been speaking with the police officers that had been called when Bree had come inside with a sobbing teenager who had begun to spill her story. It had only taken a few minutes for him to realize they were dealing with a victim of human trafficking and they needed more help than he and Bree knew how to give. Once Megan had gone into the back with Lucretia, who had been happy to play momma hen to the young girl, they'd made the call to the police.

"They've contacted Megan's mother in Memphis and she's headed to the downtown Nashville police station," Knox said when he pulled Bree into the hallway.

"I know. I talked to her mother after Megan talked to her. She needs to be taken to a hospital for an exam, but I haven't been able to bring myself to mention that yet. She's so fragile right now, Knox. Her mother says this was the first time she had run away. The first time she's done anything like that. They had a fight about a boy who had been hanging around the park where she skateboarded." Bree took a deep breath before she looked up at Knox with what could only be described as murder in her eyes. "The boy was a twenty-two-year-old man who was hooked up with other human traffickers. It was all a setup."

Knox's arm came around Bree as her whole body shook with anger. "She's only seventeen. She should feel safe to go to the park and skateboard."

Knox was afraid that the young girl might never feel safe again. "From what the officers told me, it sounds like Megan's mother will make sure she gets the help she needs."

One of the officers came out from where she had gone to talk to the young girl and handed both him and Bree a card. "We're going to take Megan downtown to meet with our human trafficking officers. She's got a lot of information that they will find helpful. She's willing to talk with them, but she wants Ms. Lucretia to go along with her. The team might have questions for you, too."

Knox, along with Bree, offered to help in any way they could. While Bree went to say goodbye to Megan and help Lucretia gather her things, Knox pulled the officer over to the side. "Is there any chance that someone followed her here? Do I need to worry about the safety of the office?"

"That's one of the reasons I gave you my card. From what Megan says, she was sent here by one of the traffickers to obtain birth control pills. If you see anything suspicious, please call."

The officer's words made Knox feel sick. He hoped that the information Megan had would help to put the traffickers away, where they belonged. If not, there'd be another girl, in another park, and that one might not have the courage to do what Megan had done.

The young girl came down the hall, Lucretia following close behind her. When the girl hesitated at the door, one of the officers got in front of her while the other followed behind them. Bree pressed a note in the girl's hand before the officer opened the door and they walked out.

"What was that?" he asked.

"I gave her my number, in case she needs something. Or if she just wants to talk." A beeper on Bree's phone went off. "I'm running behind. Ally went home with a friend today, but I don't want to be late picking her up."

Knox watched her reach into her pocket and pull out the bag holding the paternity test. "Can you drop this off for me?"

Knox reached for the bag and Bree's hand closed around his.

"I can't imagine what Megan's mother is feeling right now. She's been going through hell for two weeks wondering if her daughter was even alive. I know we have a lot going on right now, but the most important thing is Ally is safe. And I know no matter what happens with these results, she'll still be safe."

"You're right. No matter what happens with these re-sults," Knox said, "there is nothing more important than that Ally stays safe."

CHAPTER EIGHT

BREE LISTENED TO Ally chatter about her day at school as she began to mix the pancake batter. With only two more days left before summer break, Ally and her friends were getting more and more excited with plans for their time off. Bree, on the other hand, was already worried about how she was going to get someone to watch Ally on the nights she and Lori took call at the hospital. But most of all Bree was worried about the email that she had received from the lab that afternoon with the results of the paternity test.

"Is Knox going to be here soon?" Ally asked again. Ever since Bree had told her niece that she had invited Knox over for pancakes, the little girl had run back and forth from the front window to the kitchen.

Bree looked at the clock on the stove; she was getting anxious, too. Knowing that the information in the email could change both of their lives, she kept glancing over at her laptop as if the thing could open itself and spew out the information. Not that she was ready for the results on the paternity test.

While she wanted to know the truth about Ally's father, Bree knew that it could change everything about her and Ally's life. Knox had made it clear that his priority was Ally, but what did that really mean?

Bree looked around the tiny house that she had made into a home for her and Ally. It wasn't even theirs. She had been renting it month to month, not knowing where she would be settling once she got her midwifery certification. Would Knox see all the work and the love for Ally that she had put into the home? Or would he see the tiny, outdated place as something not good enough for the granddaughter of Gail and Charles Collins? He'd been brought up on a ranch that was bigger than the whole suburb where Bree had grown up.

Ally had just rushed back into the room when the doorbell finally rang. Jumping up and down with more energy than she should have had that late in the day, her niece raced back toward the door. "I've got it."

Bree forced herself not to run to the door alongside her niece. She told herself that she was anxious to see Knox because she was anxious to read the email with him. But she had been just as excited to see him every time they had passed in the halls of the Legacy Clinic that day. Something had changed between them since the day she had shared with him the truth about Ally. For the first time there had been no secrets between the two of them. She'd admitted her guilt and her fears and he'd admitted his own struggles when he was younger. If the two of them didn't have the results of the paternity test hanging over them, Bree thought that maybe the two of them might have had a chance to find something deeper.

But those results could be the very thing that destroyed that chance.

"Look what Dr. Knox brought," Ally said as Knox followed her into the kitchen carrying a large carton of chocolate milk, along with a bottle of wine.

"Is the chocolate milk for me?" Bree asked him, then looked down to Ally.

"He said it's for me, but you can have a glass," Ally said, reaching for it.

Bree turned back to the stove and began to pour the batter on the griddle. "It will definitely go with your dinner."

"It's Wednesday, so it's pancake night. Do you like pancakes?" Ally asked as she and Knox took a stool at the counter.

"I love pancakes. My mom's cook, Ms. Jenkins, makes them for breakfasts whenever I spend the night at my parents' house."

"You don't live with your mom?" Ally asked before jumping down and running over to where the dishes were kept.

"No. I have a house of my own. Like your aunt Bree."

Ally came back with the dishes and then ran back to get the utensils, explaining, "It's my job to set the table. Aunt Bree says we have to share the chores."

"That sounds like a good plan. Sharing is important," Knox said, his tone as serious as her niece's.

"So I guess the two of you can share these pancakes," Bree said as she took two plates and put a pancake on each of them. She placed bacon from the pile she had cooked earlier on each plate then brought them back to the counter. "This should get you started."

Bree listened to their conversation as she finished, then went to sit beside them at the kitchen counter that also acted as their dining table. Occasionally, she would join in, but mostly she just listened, enjoying the sound of her niece's laughter and the patience in which Knox answered all the little girl's questions.

It would have been a perfect meal if she didn't have the DNA test results weighing on her. She forced each bite of pancake down to her nervous stomach, until it protested.

"I'll do the dishes," Knox said when the last pancake had been eaten.

"You don't have to do that," Bree protested. "You're our guest tonight."

"And sometimes guests help with dishes. It's sharing, right, Ally?"

'I can help, too," Ally said as she started to take the dishes off the counter and carry them to the sink.

"Me and Knox will do the dishes. You need to go take a shower and get ready for bed," Bree said, preparing herself for the child's nightly complaints when it came to bedtime.

"Can we read tonight?" Ally asked.

"We'll see. Remember last night you took too long in the shower and we didn't have time to read." And Bree had felt guilty because it had been she who had been too tired to read that night, not Ally.

It seemed every day was getting shorter and shorter.

Each night she climbed into bed making a list of everything she needed to accomplish the next day, but it didn't seem as if she ever caught up. Between working at the two clinics, taking care of Ally and then working weekends at the bar, she never had a moment free. Add in the sleepless nights where she went from scared of what would happen with the results of the paternity to fanciful dreams of Knox kissing her again, and she was emotionally and physically drained.

"She'll be in there a while if you want us to check the email," Bree said, taking a plate from Knox and adding it to the sink.

"How about we wait until after we get these done?" Knox said as he picked up a towel.

"It's okay if you're nervous," Bree said. "I know I am."

"I'm not nervous, I'm terrified," Knox said. "Part of me wants to know the truth, while the other part worries that I'm not ready for it."

"Why is that?" she asked, though she could understand how he felt. She wanted to ask him then what his plans would be if Ally was his, while at the same time she didn't want to know what he would say.

Because unlike Knox, she was already convinced she knew what the results would be. Her sister might have changed over the last years while they'd been apart, but she didn't think Brittany would have lied about her baby's father. Why would she lie to Bree? It wouldn't have made sense.

"I'm just afraid of messing things up. My parents weren't always the best. They had a lot going on with their careers when they had me. I felt I was just an afterthought sometimes. They mostly hired staff to take care of me instead of spending time with me themselves. I'm not blaming them. The music business is rough to break in to, as I'm sure you already know. Once you get to the top, it's even harder to remain there. They did the best they could, I'm sure..."

While he said the words convincingly enough, she wasn't sure how much of it he truly believed. Families were complicated. She and her sister were a good example of that.

"I think fame and fortune change people. I know my mom changed her whole focus on life from being my mom to being me and Britt's manager. I would never want that for my child. I missed the mom I had before, the one who cared more about my everyday life than about whether I'd sung that note perfectly in practice." Bree paused with a half-washed dish in her hand, then let out a short laugh. "Don't I sound so high and mighty. The truth is, it's a struggle every day to keep my focus on Ally. I've spent most of her life working weekends to pay the bills and attending classes during the week. Some days I wonder if it was worth all the time I've missed with her. Even when I had a couple years of working in the hospital before I started midwifery school, I was working extra to pay off my college loans."

"I've seen how the two of you get along. Ally knows she's an important part of your life. You two are like a team. That's something special. I wish I'd had that with my parents. I think that's one of the reasons that my mom wants grandchildren so badly. She wants to do it right this time. And if I'm Ally's father, I want to do it right the first time. I don't want to look back like she does and see I did all the wrong things. I'll already be starting out behind."

"When Ally was born, I was only twenty-one. Suddenly, I had a baby to look after and a funeral to plan. I was drowning in grief while also trying to figure out my new life. But then one night I looked down at Ally and saw her looking up at me. I promised her then that I would be the best aunt I could be. I haven't been perfect, Knox, I know that. But I want you to know that I've always done my best."

She turned off the water and dried her hands. "I don't know how this is going to work out. If you aren't Ally's father, I will have to decide if I want to pursue finding out who is. I'll be honest. I don't think that's something I'm going to do. At least, not until she's older."

"But is that fair to Ally or to her father?" Knox asked.

Bree headed to the small sitting area where she had left her computer. "I don't know. I didn't have a choice in telling you. Not with the information I had from Brittany. And not now after I got to know that you aren't the person I thought you were. I told you about Ally as much for her sake as for yours. I promised that I would be truthful to her, and keeping this from her isn't the right thing for me to do."

She opened the laptop and began to sign in to her email account. "But I'll be honest. If you had wanted to walk away after I told you about Ally, I would have been okay with that."

He looked at her and she could already feel the crack forming on her heart. Because she knew the man Knox was now. He wouldn't walk away no matter how much more simple it would make both their lives.

"Open the email, Bree. I'm not going anywhere."

Knox sat down beside Bree as she opened the email from the lab. This was it. His life could change forever at this moment. Looking over at Bree, he had to admit to himself that his life had already changed. Bree had opened up the possibility of a new world to him. One that he hadn't known he wanted. Already he was trying to figure out how he was going to fit a little girl into his life as a traveling doctor, always moving from town to town. And every time he pictured his new life with Ally, Bree was always there, too. Right beside him. And that was just one more thing that scared him. He knew she was scared. She'd raised Ally alone for eight years and now he was there threatening the life she'd made for them.

"Okay, here it is," Bree said as she hovered over the results, her finger hesitating before tapping it.

As the email opened, Bree reached for his hand, the connection to her soothing in a way he couldn't explain. She had made it sound like the two of them were adversaries, but still, she wanted him beside her. He tightened his grip, hoping to give back some of the comfort she so readily gave to him.

They read the email silently, but together. When they

had both finished, Bree shut the laptop, then turned to him. "My sister might have had a lot of faults, but lying wasn't one of them."

Knox just nodded his head. He was so full of emotions that he couldn't speak. He had a daughter.

The sound of little bare feet slapping against the wooden floors seemed to be the only sound in the house. Bree let go of his hand and moved away just moments before Ally ran into the room, her damp hair flying around her face. She dropped down on the couch between him and Bree, the smile on her face disappearing as she looked between the two of them. "What's wrong?"

"Nothing is wrong," Bree said, before looking at Knox. "It's just as it should be."

The words struck Knox like a battering ram, opening his eyes to what was really there before him. Ally was his daughter. His daughter. Wow. His mother was going to need sedatives when she got the news.

And when was he going to tell her? It wasn't right not to share the news, but didn't Ally need to be told first? And how were they going to tell Ally? Because it had to be both of them telling her. That, he knew.

"Why don't you tell Knox good-night and go get your book out for us to read?"

"Can Dr. Knox read the book with me?" Ally asked, looking from her aunt to him. His chest was suddenly tight as emotions he'd never felt before began to surface. His little girl wanted him to read to her? Was it possible that she felt the connection between the two of them without being told? Was that even possible? The two of them had gotten along well since the moment Bree had introduced the two of them. Knox didn't know everything about Bree's life before they started working at the clinic together, but wasn't it more likely that Ally just hadn't had many men in her life? Bree was very focused on Ally and her career. It could be that like him, she hadn't had time for a serious romantic involvement, and having a man at their home was just something different.

"If he'd like to do that, it's fine with me," Bree told her niece before looking over at him.

Knox didn't miss the pool of tears that were forming in her eyes. While he'd been there processing what being Ally's father meant for him and his family, what had Bree been feeling?

"Please?" Ally asked, hopping up and down on the seat next to him.

This was the first thing his daughter had asked of him. Looking into Ally's brilliant green eyes that reminded him so much of Bree's, he knew he couldn't disappoint her. "Sure, but you might have to help me with the big words."

"I can read most of them, but Aunt Bree has to help me sometimes. She can help you, too," Ally said, her face all serious with not a hint of a smile.

"I think the two of you will be fine without me," Bree said, giving her niece a watery smile. "And I've got some work to do on my computer before I go to bed."

Knox gave Bree a smile, unsure what else to do as Ally took his hand and began to pull him down the hall to her room. He and Bree had a lot to talk about, but it would all have to wait until Ally went to sleep.

A half an hour later, after reading a total of four pages before Ally had fallen asleep, he returned to the living room only to find her aunt with her own eyes closed, her hands resting on the keys of her laptop. Carefully, he removed the laptop before taking the seat next to her. Bree shifted and her head came to rest on his shoulder. But instead of waking, she seemed to settle into sleep even deeper, her lips curving into an innocent smile, so much like his daughter's.

Like his daughter's. Wasn't it weird how that thought seemed to come so easily now? An hour ago the thought of having a child was something foreign and frightening. Now it just felt...right.

Bree's eyes blinked open and she looked around the room, slowly sitting up. "Ally?"

"She was asleep before the wizard had his first dance at the ball," Knox said, staring down into Bree's sleep-drugged eyes.

"She'll be disappointed in the morning. It's one of her favorite scenes," she said, stretching and moving away from him. "Thank you for doing that."

"Thank you for letting me," he said. "Thank you for everything. I don't know how I can ever repay you for taking care of Ally all these years. I don't want to think about what might have happened to her if you hadn't been there for her."

When Bree stiffened beside him, he realized he had said the wrong thing. "I don't mean to insult you. I know she's your niece and you've taken care of her because you love her."

"She's not just my niece, Knox. She's my child in every way except that I didn't give birth to her. We're all the family the two of us have had. Until now," Bree said as she moved away from him, then let out a deep sigh. "I know we have a lot to discuss, but I think it would be best to wait until another day. We're both tired and there's a lot for both of us to take in now that we both know the truth."

"Bree, I don't want to make this hard on you," Knox started, then stopped. Of course this was hard on Bree. That test had changed her life, too. But not all change was bad. In his way of seeing things, this could be a good thing for both of them. He just had to give her time to see that.

Pulling her feet up onto the couch and curling into a protective ball, she looked so small and defenseless. He tried to think of something to say. It was as if all the tension that had existed between the two of them before they had begun to work together had suddenly resurfaced. They'd come so far and now it was more important than ever that they got along.

But she was right, it was late and they were both expected at the clinic the next day. Standing, he looked down at her. "We'll talk tomorrow."

"Tomorrow," Bree said, nodding her head. "We can both talk tomorrow."

CHAPTER NINE

WHILE KNOX TRIED to catch Bree between patients the next day, they were both busy from the start of the day until Lucretia put the closed sign out on the office door. Bree had mentioned earlier in the week that there were only a few days left before school was out for the summer break. He expected things would be hectic till then, but he wanted to discuss when, and how, they were going to let Ally know that he was her father. It was the *how* that worried him the most. He wasn't equipped for a "how I met your mother" type of conversation with an eight-year-old.

He'd just finished seeing his last patient of the day when Bree stepped out from the exam room with her own patient. He waited while she handed the patient a prescription along with some samples before he joined her.

"And this is Dr. Collins," Bree said, introducing him to a young woman who looked to be about Bree's age. "This is Kelly. She's just moved to town and needed a refill on her birth control until she can get set up with a primary doctor."

"It's so great that this clinic is open for walk-ins.

There's nothing like this where I'm from and my insurance doesn't start for another two weeks. I've got three little ones at home. I didn't want to take a chance on adding to that number."

While Bree and Kelly discussed things from potty training to the best time to change from a bottle to a cup, Knox listened. He'd missed both of those steps with Ally. He'd missed all the firsts. First steps. First words. Even the first day of school. He couldn't blame Bree for any of that; she had only been looking out for his daughter. But still, he wished he'd been there. He was sure Bree would be glad to share baby pictures, but it wasn't the same as being there. He'd just have to make a point of being there for all the other things, though how was he going to do that? He'd spent the past few years traveling from clinic to clinic. He and Bree had a lot of things to discuss.

"Well, that's the last one," Lucretia said, locking the door behind Bree's patient. "I think we might have set a record today. I know Dr. Reynolds will be impressed when he returns and sees the numbers. We've been able to see almost twice as many patients since you brought Bree here. Maybe he'll be able to get some other midwives in to help."

Knox had kept Dean Reynolds up-to-date with the running of the clinic through regular text messages and when he'd mentioned bringing a midwife resident in, the other doctor had thought it a great idea. Neither of them had expected it to be this successful. Knox had especially been concerned after the way Bree had initially reacted to Dr. Warner's suggestion that she spend time at the clinic.

* * *

"I'll mention it to my preceptor and my nurse counselor at the college," Bree said. "I've enjoyed the work here and I've gotten a lot of experience I wouldn't have gotten otherwise. I'm sure there are more midwives that would be interested."

"I don't guess I can talk you into staying," Lucretia said.

"I don't know what I'll be doing once I finish my residency. But if I'm in Nashville, I'll certainly try to volunteer a couple times a month," Bree said. The alarm on her watch went off, and she slid the straps of her backpack on. She was about to make her escape before they had a chance to talk.

"Do you have a moment to discuss…a few things?" Knox asked, aware that Lucretia would overhear anything that he said to Bree.

"I'm sorry, but Ally's class is having an art exhibit this afternoon at the school and I promised I would be there."

Knox was surprised at the hurt her words caused. Shouldn't he have been invited now that Bree knew for certain that he was Ally's father? He decided then and there that he wasn't going to miss another day of his daughter's life. "I'd love to see Ally's artwork. We can talk on the way there."

While Bree hesitated, Knox headed for the door. The hurt he felt from not being invited was turning into anger, something that was very rare for him. He fought against it as they exited the building as neither of them said a word. Bree's car door had barely shut when he let go of the words he had been holding back. "Why didn't you tell me Ally had something going on at school? I thought I made it clear that I wanted to be a part of her life."

"It's just a bunch of pictures drawn by a class of eight-year-olds. I didn't think you would be interested," Bree said, her eyes fixed on the windshield in front of her as she started the car.

"But it's my eight-year-old's pictures," Knox said, then realized he sounded like an eight-year-old himself.

Bree looked over at him then; her bright green eyes held none of the sparkle he was used to. "I'm sorry. I didn't think about inviting you. Like I said, it's just a bunch of pictures that they've drawn throughout the year."

"Is it a big deal to Ally?" Knox asked, knowing the answer. "I remember all the school activities that my parents missed while they were out touring. I remember the disappointment of not having anyone there for me."

"Ally isn't you, Knox. I've been to almost every activity she's had at school for the last three years." She looked at her watch, then turned off the car. "I realize this has all been a shock to you. We both have a lot to process. I promise that I'll be better at communicating with you while we work things out, but you using words like *my daughter* isn't going to help. Ally is mine, too."

"Of course, Ally is yours, too," Knox said, his hands instinctively running through his hair. He was messing all of this up with Bree. He didn't want things to be this way. Not for Ally. And not for him and Bree, either. They both wanted what was best for Ally. They needed to be united or this could turn into one of those ugly battles adults get into over their children.

And maybe that meant giving them both some time to come to terms with what this new reality would mean for the two of them was a good idea. "I'll admit that finding out Ally is my daughter has brought up some old feelings I probably need to deal with. I know you've been there for Ally and I shouldn't compare my childhood to hers."

"How about, for now, I promise to include you in Ally's life while we sort out things between the two of us?" Bree asked. "We can enjoy today and then I think we need to deal with things between the two of us before we move forward with telling Ally anything."

"I can live with that. I think seeing us together more would be good for Ally, too. It would give her more security when we tell her about me being her father. Get her used to me being around on a regular basis. Does that work for you?" He wanted to move forward with telling Ally about him, but he understood that he and Bree had to do it together. He'd have to be patient.

And he'd enjoyed spending time with Bree and Ally before he'd even known about the possibility of being Ally's father. Now spending time with them would mean even more. He also hoped that working out things between them would also include more kisses like the one they had shared at the ranch. He had to believe that her response to him that day meant she had felt the same magnetic pull that he had felt almost from the moment he'd met her. That wasn't magically going to go away just because of the results of the paternity test.

"I can work with that," Bree said, restarting the car. "The most important thing is for us to make this as easy on Ally as possible. That means both of us taking into consideration what is best for her in whatever decisions we make."

Was she unknowingly answering Knox's thoughts about her words and the situation that they were both in now? Was that her way of telling him that they needed to ignore what had been building between them? If so, he would have to make it a point to change her mind. Because just like things would never go back to the way they were before he learned he was Ally's father, he didn't want things to go back to the way they had been before he had found Bree.

Bree watched Knox as he went from picture to picture with Ally pulling him down the line of drawings that had been hung on her classroom walls. He smiled and commented on each picture as if it were hanging in a New York City museum. It should have surprised her, and it would have two months ago when she had thought of him as a spoiled rich kid who had gone through life ruining young girls' lives, just like she had imagined that he had done to Brittany. But now that she knew him? No, it didn't surprise her at all. What did surprise her was the way her heart hammered every time he turned to look at her and gave her that wicked smile of his that sent shivers running up her spine and heat settling in places where it shouldn't be. How could she have such a response to a man whom she'd given the power to take away the child she'd raised? Shouldn't her heart see the danger it was in? Well, maybe her heart did, but her body wasn't listening to anything it had to say.

"Look, look! Those are my pictures there," Ally said, dragging Knox down to where her pictures hung. Bree recognized one of them as being the picture her niece had drawn of her family. "That's a picture of me and Aunt Bree in front of our house. And this is a picture of my mommy in heaven. My teacher helped me draw it because my friends asked me why I didn't have a mommy or daddy and I didn't know what to say."

Bree pushed back against the pain of seeing an eight-year-old's idea of what her mother would look like as an angel. Sometimes she felt very inadequate in filling her sister's place as Ally's mom. It was something she had dealt with from the first moment she'd held Ally in her arms. Mostly, she had learned to ignore the feeling that she wasn't enough. It wasn't that she wanted to replace her sister. There would always be a place in both Ally's and Bree's hearts for Brittany. But looking at the picture of a stick figure woman with hair the color of Bree's and eyes that matched hers, too, Bree could feel the loss Ally felt and she had never known how to fill it.

As if Knox understood that this was something she was sensitive about, he reached back and took her hand, pulling her up beside the two of them. Then he did something that was totally unexpected. Taking out his phone, then smiling at Ally's teacher, who had been hovering around the parents and students, he waved her over to the three of them. "Do you mind taking a picture for me?"

Ally's teacher took the phone as Knox turned Bree toward the camera while draping his arm across her shoulder and positioning Ally between the two of them. If Bree's smile was a little watery when the teacher handed the phone back to him, he didn't comment.

"This is Aunt Bree's boyfriend, Dr. Knox," Ally said, introducing him to her teacher.

"I...ah..." Bree tried to get the denial out of her lips, but the words were jumbled up inside her brain as she tried to recover from her niece's words. Looking over at Knox for help, she watched as he introduced himself and shook the woman's hand, never once denying Ally's statement. By the time Bree could form a half-witted sentence, the teacher had moved on to another student.

When Knox suggested that they stop at the same pizza place they had visited before, Ally immediately set to getting Bree to agree. It was easy for Bree to see why Ally thought of Knox as her *boyfriend*. Bree had spent more time out with Knox in the past three weeks than she'd spent with any other man since she'd had Ally.

As they ate, she watched as Ally and Knox laughed at a show on the screen above their table. She had never noticed before, but the two of them had a similar laugh. One of those whole-body laughs where their grins were wide and their eyes crinkled in the corners. She couldn't help but laugh, too, even though she wasn't watching the show. She only had eyes for the two of them as they clowned around with each other. With everything in her heart, she wished she could freeze that moment. There were so many things that would be changing soon, for all of them. But she didn't want to think about that tonight. Tonight she was going to just enjoy them being together like this. If a part of her was pretending that the three of them were just a normal family out for the night, who did that hurt?

When Knox looked over at her, his eyes shining with happiness, she picked up her glass of wine and took a sip before giving him a smile. He was a good man. An honest man. A caring man. One that worked in under-privileged communities when he could work in any OB/GYN clinic in the country. And it was already clear that he loved Ally just as much as she did. What more could she ask for as a father for her niece?

That was why after he carried the sleeping little girl into her bedroom and helped Bree get her tucked into bed for the night, she decided that he deserved some one-on-one time with his daughter.

"I've got the early-evening shift at the bar Saturday night. Would you like to watch Ally for me?" she asked as they stopped at the door.

"Of course, I'll keep Ally. What time do you want me here?" Knox said. It almost hurt Bree to see how happy her request made him. It was like giving a starving man a piece of bread. He'd been like this since the moment he'd found out Ally was his.

"If you could be here at four-thirty I can make it in by five. I'm only working till eleven. I take the early-evening shift so my usual babysitter isn't too late getting home. She just lives across the street, but she's older and her husband doesn't like her out any later than midnight." Bree had always thought it was more that Fran's husband couldn't sleep himself until his wife came home. Not that she minded. She knew that she had been lucky to have so many people to help her out with Ally over the years.

"I'll be here," Knox said. He opened his mouth to say something else, then stopped.

"What is it?" she asked. "If you have something else planned, it's okay."

"No. I'm not on call this weekend. There's nothing I'd rather do Saturday night."

He stepped closer to her and placed a light kiss on her lips, lingering there for only a second, resting his forehead against hers. Before she could react, he'd stepped away. "Thank you for this evening."

She watched as he made his way to where a car waited for him and she wondered what he would have said if she'd had the nerve to ask him to stay the night instead of taking a hired service back to the office to get his own car. If the look in his eyes before he'd left was any indication, she was pretty sure he would have stayed. And she would have been glad to let him.

CHAPTER TEN

Knox looked around what had been Bree's orderly living room. He hadn't known what to expect, but the stack of books and pile of games that lay open around the room wasn't it. Though Ally had never appeared to be a low-energy child, she'd been more energetic than usual. Maybe it had been the ice cream he'd brought for dessert. Or the sprinkles that they'd added when Ally had shown him where her aunt hid them.

Looking at the clock, he knew he had only moments to get the mess cleaned up before Bree arrived. He didn't want to give her the impression that he couldn't handle taking care of his eight-year-old daughter. He needed her to see him as a capable parent. He had a lot to make up to both Bree and Ally. He didn't know how he was going to do it, but he would spend the rest of his life trying.

As the front door opened, he stacked the last of the board games together. Turning, he saw that the smiling Bree that had left just hours ago now looked like she couldn't take another step. The laughter that had been in her eyes when she'd been warning Knox of all the ways Ally would try to escape her bedtime was gone. Her mascara was just smudges under her eyes now and there was nothing left of the pretty pink lipstick that he'd been thinking about since the moment she'd walked out.

"Hard night?" he asked. He hadn't made it a secret that he didn't like her working as much as she was, but he knew she wouldn't appreciate his concern. He would have to be very careful when he approached the subject.

"It was bachelorette party central tonight. There had to be at least ten of them that came in. The place was packed," Bree said, landing on the couch before slipping her shoes off.

Knox watched as she wiggled her toes back and forth as if trying to return the circulation to them. He sat down on the rug in front of her and pulled off her simple white socks and began to massage the pale pink polished toes.

"What are you doing?" Bree asked. He looked up to see her eyes closed, and the muscles of her tired face relaxing.

"My father used to do this for my mother when they'd had a long night on stage. She said it helped her unwind. Is it working?"

Instead of answering, she let out a moan, then stretched her legs out farther, arching her back and burrowing into the couch. Something inside him awakened with that sound. His mind went to places he'd been avoiding since the day they'd kissed at the ranch. When she arched her back and burrowed deeper into the couch, he forced himself to concentrate on what he was doing. Then his hands moved up to the calves of her legs and the tension in her body disappeared. His hands reached the backs of her knees and he looked up to see Bree watching him, her eyelids barely opened. When she didn't tell him to stop, he continued.

Unfortunately, his own body was tightening with each stroke of his hands across her soft skin. Desire ran through his system, the heat of it flooding his veins. His heartbeat drummed to a different beat in his chest, each beat becoming faster and faster. What had started as a way to comfort Bree had turned on him. His body was now as tight as a guitar string. He didn't know when he'd ever been this aroused.

Then his hands slid higher, brushing against the tattered hem of her denim shorts, and Bree let out a gasp before arching her back again.

"Do you want me to stop?" he asked as he came up on his knees, his eyes even with hers.

"No, please don't stop," she said, her hands tentatively coming up to rest on his chest. She bit her lower lip then looked up at him, an innocence and trust in her eyes that had his body going into overdrive. Bree had always been a woman of secrets to him, always holding back something even as she smiled and laughed and looked so innocent. He wanted to know all her secrets tonight, especially the ones her body held.

He moved over her and slowly lowered himself until their lips touched. She tasted of sunshine and honey and when her tongue welcomed his, he couldn't resist the pleasure there. They tangled, released and then tangled again, his mouth wanting more and more as it caught each moan she gave him.

When her hands reached for the hem of his T-shirt, he scooped her up off the couch and carried her toward the bedroom. Her green eyes seemed to shine in the darkness as they left the light of the living room and headed down the hall. When her mouth moved up his neck, he had to stop and lean against the wall. "If you don't stop, we won't make it to your bed."

"Really," she said, surprise and a sweet, sexy smile dancing across her swollen lips before they returned to torturing him as they moved down to his collarbone.

"Behave," he said as he gritted his teeth and forced his feet to start moving again. Only the presence of his daughter in the room down the hall kept him moving forward.

He made it to the door of her room, pushed it open and unceremoniously dumped her in the middle of the bed. He finished stripping his shirt off and then paused at the sight of Bree staring at him. When she came up on her knees and put her hands on his belt buckle, his whole body went rock-hard.

"I don't know exactly how to do all this, but I think I can handle it," she said. Her hand began to undo his belt while her lips trailed soft kisses down his chest. What was she saying? That she was innocent? That couldn't be; she was only four years younger than him. He was suddenly out of his depth.

"Are you saying that you're a virgin?" he asked, his head swimming from the possibility.

Bree's hands stilled and she sat back on her heels. "Is that a problem?"

There was a vulnerability in her voice that shook loose every protective instinct in his body. "No, sweetheart, it's not a problem. It's a privilege. I just need to know. I don't want to hurt you."

"Okay," she said, her hands less sure as they fumbled with his belt now. His hands covered hers and he bent down to kiss her. The desire that had almost consumed them earlier returned as he nibbled at her lips until she was moaning again.

While this would be a first for Bree, it would also be a first for him. The women he'd been involved with before had always been as experienced as him. Even his first lover, one of his parents' crew members and a few years older, had been skilled in the art of making love. He wanted to make this special for both of them, but especially for her. He knew in his heart that this was a memory he would always treasure. He wanted to have a memory just as precious as she was.

When Bree finished removing his belt, he let her unzip his jeans, but stilled her hand when it closed around him, wrapping his around hers. Her grip tightened and he moaned as he locked her eyes onto his, his hips rocking against her hand. "This is what you do to me, Bree."

As his control began to crumble, he removed her hands and raised them over her head. "Stay like this."

He thought she'd protest, but she kept her arms up as he peeled her T-shirt off her body, uncovering a pale pink bra that displayed softly rounded breasts. Her skin was a pale pink that reminded him of peaches and cream and he knew it would taste just as sweet. Unable to help himself, he bent and licked the top of each breast. The shiver that ran through her body, transferring itself to him... His body shaking, he held himself in check. He removed her bra, his mind taking in each curve. He laid her down and undid her shorts, while his lips sprinkled kisses over her breasts then down her abdomen. Time stood still for a moment as he spread her legs. When he looked into her eyes and saw not only desire, but trust, too, his heart filled his chest with an emotion he had never shared with another person.

"Do you know how special you are, Bree Rogers? Do you have any idea what you have done to me?" he asked.

"I just know that I want you," Bree whispered back to him. "Is that enough?"

He didn't answer her back. For now it would have to be enough. But when he bent his head and tasted her most private places, he knew that this night with Bree would never be enough for him.

Bree's mind tried to wrap around the reality of the moment while her body flooded with sensations that it had never experienced. Finding Knox waiting for her when she'd come home had seemed so right tonight. And when his hands had begun their lazy exploration of her legs as he'd massaged each aching spot, she'd been overcome with a desire for more as every nerve ending in her body called out to be touched by him. She'd arched into his touch as her body had cried out for more. Just more. But of what?

When his lips had touched her, she'd thought, *This is it. This is what I need.* But still, that hadn't been enough.

Now, as she lay there with all her innocence exposed to him, the desire for something more was almost painful. He lowered his head and gently kissed the inside of her thigh, and her body almost bucked off the bed. Never had her body been so sensitive. She bit her lip as his lips lazily moved inside her thigh. And then his hands parted her and her breath caught as his tongue raked across her center.

Her hands clutched his head, her fingers tangling in his curls, and her body came off the bed as she was suddenly inundated with sensations that wanted to overwhelm her. It felt like every nerve ending she had was too sensitive. Knox's hands joined her mouth as he left no part of her unscathed as he tormented her with a pleasure that built until she wanted to scream. She tried to tell him it was too much, but the words died in her throat as the pleasure inside her body began to build. As the orgasm hit her, she grabbed on to it, embracing it. Her world shattered and she knew everything about her had suddenly changed.

When her mind righted itself, she opened her eyes to find Knox staring down at her. With her brain still jumbled, she could only get out the most important of words. "More."

"Are you sure?" Knox asked, his face set in hard lines,

his body hard against hers, his breaths coming just as fast as hers.

"Please," she said as she lifted a hand to his cheek. He wouldn't understand that she had never been with another man because there had never been one she'd wanted to share her first time with, until now. "I want this. With you."

Even as relaxed as she was, her body tightened as she watched him roll on a condom he'd produced from his jeans. He was as beautiful a man undressed as he was dressed. Uncertainty filled her, along with fear that she'd disappoint him. Of course, she knew the mechanics and she'd read enough on the subject to know what to expect.

But when he entered her, so gently, she found a new desire as he filled her. If there was pain, the pleasure overrode it. And when he began to move inside her, she let her body respond, holding nothing back from him.

As a new climax, this one even stronger than the one before, began to build inside her, she opened her eyes and found his eyes fixed on hers. A scream tore through her and his mouth sealed over hers as they both rode the orgasm out together. Yes, her world was definitely never going to be the same again.

"I have to go," Knox whispered in Bree's ear, brushing her hair aside as he applied a soft kiss to her neck.

Bree opened her eyes and saw the clock. It was almost five. Her mind tried to remember the day. Was she at the clinic or the hospital today? No. She'd worked the night before. Before…

Her eyes popped open and she took in her surroundings. She was in her bed. The sun had begun to come up, casting shadows between the dark curtains on her windows, and she could see a pile of clothes scattered across the wooden plank floors.

She'd worked last night at the bar and when she'd come home Knox had been there. More memories of the night returned, explaining why she was in her bed and why Knox was bending over her.

She'd slept with Knox. She wouldn't regret it. It had been perfect. Knox had been perfect. Not that she was really surprised. The attraction between them, though she'd tried to ignore it, had been growing for a while.

But still, he was the father of her niece: the one person who could take her away from Bree. How would it affect Ally if she ended up involved with him? And shouldn't she feel some kind of guilt for the fact that her sister had once been, though shortly, involved with Knox? It was a complication that they didn't need in a relationship that was already complicated both emotionally and legally. It was just too bad that her body and her heart hadn't come up with that information before things had gotten this far.

There was so much between them that had to be settled before they could address any of this. But instead of sitting up and facing all of it, she closed her eyes and pretended to fall back off to sleep. When Knox kissed her forehead before leaving, she curled deeper into the bed covers. Maybe if she buried herself deep enough, she could just this once enjoy her memories of the night before she had to face the consequences that would come with the day.

CHAPTER ELEVEN

Monday morning, Bree walked into Legacy Women's Clinic cautiously. She'd never had the experience that other women talked about as far as the awkward mornings when you saw someone you'd slept with. There'd been no walks of shame for her. While the other college girls had been hooking up with guys, she'd been raising her niece. She didn't know how to handle things like this. She didn't want to embarrass herself or Knox by making too much of the fact that they had slept together. But how did she do that when what they'd shared had been earth-shattering to her? How did she act all nonchalant when she knew just seeing him would bring up memories of the night they had shared?

When the first thing she saw was Knox where he stood deep in a conversation with Sable, the office manager, she did the first thing she could think of. She ducked into the first door she could find. It wasn't until she heard someone clearing her voice that she realized it was Lori's office. Turning, she found her mentor, along with the practice's other midwife, Sky, staring at her.

"Sorry, I just…" Bree tried to think of some excuse that would have her interrupting the two of them. Before her brain cells supplied her with anything that sounded plausible, Sky went to the door and cracked it open.

"Well, well," Sky said, shutting the door behind her and giving Bree a questioning look before looking over at Lori. "Since I'm thinking it would be very unlikely that you are trying to avoid the office manager, it seems our new midwife is avoiding Nashville's famous bad boy."

"That's not who he is anymore," Bree said, realizing too late that taking up for Knox was the last thing she should have done. "I mean, I don't think it's fair to judge him by what he did when he was a kid."

"Oh, she's got it bad, Lori," Sky said.

Bree felt the blush as it crept up her face. Bree knew she was only teasing her, but the midwife had hit too close to the truth.

"Stop teasing her, Sky. It wasn't that long ago that you were mooning around over Jared."

"I never," Sky said, then stopped. "Okay, maybe I did."

When Lori's eyes turned back to her, Bree wanted to slide under the door and take her chances with being cornered by Knox even though she still didn't know she'd feel uncomfortable seeing him there after what they'd shared. How did people do this? It wasn't that she was embarrassed that they'd had sex. Or that she felt they'd done something wrong. They were both consenting adults. It had just seemed so intimate. And he knew she had been a virgin. She'd bared so much of herself to him. Been so intimate when she normally held back so much. Maybe the word for what she felt was *shy*?

"When me and Jack set it up for you to work at the clinic, you were very adamant about not wanting to work with Knox. I think your exact words were 'I just don't find him particularly likeable.' I take it that has changed? Did the two of you kiss and make up?"

Bree's face got even hotter. There had been a time when she and her sister had teased each other unmercifully like this. She missed the closeness that she'd shared with her twin. It had been years since she'd had someone to tease her.

"Oh, my goodness, you kissed him?" Skylar said before busting out laughing.

"Sky, stop it. You're embarrassing her," Lori said before turning to Bree. "Please tell me you didn't kiss him."

When Bree didn't answer her, Lori dropped her head onto the desk. "It's all my fault. I feel like I threw you to the wolves."

"Okay, the two of you need to stop," Bree said.

"I'm sorry," Lori said, lifting her head. "We shouldn't have teased you. But in all seriousness, I don't want you to be hurt. I know Knox has changed a lot since he went into medicine. The work he does in the rural areas is tremendous. But what do you really know about him?"

Bree almost laughed. The two of them had no idea. Not that she could explain all of that to them. His being Ally's father would eventually come out. There would be no way to keep that news private. It was even possible that it would be reported in the media at some point because of his parents, which could bring up the story of Brittany's death. She and Knox would have to find a way to protect Ally from the attention if that happened. Just one more reason to make sure they told Ally about her mother and Knox carefully. The child had lost her mother suddenly; it didn't seem right that she should suddenly be faced, while unprepared, with a daddy, too.

"I'm a big girl. I can handle it," Bree told the two of them, turning toward the door. And for the first time since Knox had left her bed, she felt like she could handle it. She could handle all of it. The way her and Knox's relationship was changing, the need to find a way to explain Knox's sudden presence in his daughter's life to Ally, and even the fact that Knox could now have more rights to her niece than Bree did. Knowing him now, she felt safe that the two of them could work together to make all this work. And yes, she was even beginning to believe that she, Knox and Ally might be able to find a happy ending together.

That thought put a smile on her face that lasted throughout the day. After that, the hours went by fast as she and Lori saw mostly obstetric patients and then attended a late-afternoon delivery, which left a smiling new family with a healthy baby girl. It wasn't until she was rounding on their last postpartum patient that she saw Knox. She started toward him, then saw that he was in a deep conversation with one of the anesthesia nurses. When the woman smiled at him, Bree remembered her toothpaste-ad smile. A feeling came over Bree that she had never felt before. Possessiveness? Jealousy? A mixture of both? It wasn't a feeling she liked. While she had no claim over Knox, she also knew he wouldn't have slept with her if he was involved with someone else. That thought calmed the green-eyed monster that had wanted to come out. Instead, she managed a smile and wave as she passed the two of them in the hall, then continued to her patient's room.

She wasn't surprised when she came out to find Knox waiting for her. She'd known in her heart that he would want to see her as much as she wanted to see him. It seemed like days since she'd seen that smile of his, and seeing it made her smile, too. Why had she been so concerned that things would be awkward between them? There was no awkwardness now. Instead, there was an openness, an honesty, that had always been missing. She liked the way things were between them now better than the way things had been when she'd been keeping secrets.

"I'm glad I caught up with you. I kept missing you at the office," Knox said when he saw her. "I'd thought we'd share lunch, but you were tied up with Lori."

"It's been a busy day. Do you have a patient delivering?" she asked.

"No, I've just finished a Cesarean section. A patient with a complete previa came in bleeding," he said, falling in beside her as she started back down the hall toward the exit.

"The mom and baby?" she asked, though she knew they had to be okay or he wouldn't be standing there all relaxed.

"Both doing good, though mom is receiving her second blood transfusion now. I was going to see if you'd let me take you and Ally out to supper, but I think I'd better stay here. She's still having more bleeding than I would like. I wanted to spend some time with y'all, though."

Looking down at her watch, she saw that there was only a few minutes before her alarm would go off and she'd have to be on her way to pick Ally up at the local athletic center, which provided summer day care. "I understand. I'm about to head out to pick up Ally now. Maybe you could call later tonight?"

"I will," he said, then turned when one of the labor and delivery nurses came rushing toward him, calling his name.

"That doesn't look good. You better go. Just call me later," Bree said, waving him away when he looked back at her. She watched as Knox jogged toward the nurse then started giving orders. She heard *OR* and knew his patient wasn't doing well. There had once been a time when she'd wanted to be the doctor standing there giving orders. Tonight she was glad that it wasn't her.

Bree rushed into the county clinic pulling a slow-moving Ally by the straps of her backpack behind her.

"There you are. I wondered if you were going to show up today. I know this is your last week but it's not the time to be slacking," Lucretia said with her usual big-dog bark and her puppy-dog bite. Then Ally peeped from behind Bree. "Wait. Who is that?"

"This is Ally, my niece," Bree said. "And Ally, this is Ms. Lucretia. She works with me and Dr. Knox."

Ally gave the woman a little wave, then looked around the room. "Don't you have a TV in your waiting room?"

"When we got to Ally's summer care program there was a note that they had a water pipe burst and would be closed till it was fixed. Knox said it was okay for me to bring Ally to work. I thought maybe she could hang out in reception with you?"

"Of course, she can. I can always use a helper," Lucretia said.

"Did I hear my name?" Knox said, coming in from the back of the office. "Hey, Ally. How do you like the clinic?"

Bree watched as Ally's disappointed face changed immediately. Running across the room, the little girl threw herself against Knox. Hugging Ally, he looked up at Bree. Even with her limited experience with it, she knew that it was love she saw in Knox's eyes. But when he looked down at Ally, Bree couldn't help but wonder if all that love had been for his daughter or if, maybe, some of it had been for her.

Which was a ridiculous thing for her to even be worrying about. Why did her mind constantly go to the negative where Knox was concerned? Was it the uncertainty of where the two stood after the night they'd spent together? Probably. She lay in the bed last night waiting for his call, the whole time wondering if she was making too much of that night. And then she'd remember how happy he'd seemed when he'd seen her at the hospital before he'd rushed off to an emergency, and she'd felt better.

But when the hours without a call from him had continued to tick away, she'd been left feeling forgotten and alone. Was this what her sister had felt like?

She realized then that Ally had been talking to her. "Can we, Aunt Bree?"

Bree looked from Ally to Knox. "I'm sorry, can we what?"

"I was telling her that my mother had invited the two of you back to the ranch this Saturday. I know it's Jared and Sky's weekend on call, so you and Lori should be free." There was something in Knox's voice that said this wasn't a simple invitation. He seemed to be holding his breath as he waited for her answer. Her mother's instinct was warning her that something was up.

"How about we talk about this later? We'll have patients coming in any minute and I want to get Ally set up with some of her toys in the reception office." Bree was prepared for the disappointment and the whining that came from Ally as she began to bargain in order to secure Bree's agreement to the trip. What she wasn't prepared for was the disappointment in Knox's eyes. But when he turned and walked away, she knew that they would be discussing this later.

But when the morning rush hit and Bree went from patient to patient performing everything from Pap smears to treating abscess infections, she didn't have the time to worry about the fact that both Ally and Knox weren't happy with her. Between every patient, she checked on Ally. While she might not have been happy with her aunt, the rest of her behavior couldn't have been better. Lucretia had put her to work stapling together the handouts they supplied to the women they see to find other resources to help with housing and food. Not for the first time Bree thought how lucky she was that she'd been able to provide for Ally over the years. It hadn't been easy, but her little girl had never gone to bed hungry and she'd always had a safe place to live.

She'd just checked on Ally and was headed back to see a new patient when Knox waved her into an empty exam room.

"Can we talk for a minute?" he asked, the seriousness in his voice so different from his usual joking manner.

"I have a patient waiting," she began.

"There will always be a patient waiting. It won't take but a moment." Knox opened the door wider and she walked in.

"I wanted to talk last night, but by the time I left the hospital it was too late." When he offered her a chair, she took it. If he wanted her to be seated, he had already decided that she wasn't going to like whatever it was he wanted to say.

"The patient with the previa? How is she?" Bree asked, mainly because she had worried about the patient when she'd left the hospital, but also so she could stall Knox from saying whatever it was that she knew would change things between them.

"There was no stopping the bleeding. I had to perform a hysterectomy," Knox said. "It was their second child and they had wanted more. I hated it, but it was either that or she was going to bleed to death. I went by to see them this morning and they both know they made the right choice."

"I'm sorry that it ended that way, but I'm glad she's okay." Of course they made the right choice. The only choice they really had. Sometimes the hardest choices are the ones where there really isn't a choice. Telling you that you have a choice is just someone's way of giving you some power over the situation, when truly your power has been taken away. Bree had faced those choices in her own life. Right now she felt that she was about to face another one of them.

"I wanted to talk to you about Ally. I think she's ready for us to tell her that I'm her father." When Bree started to interrupt him, Knox stopped her. "Can you honestly tell me that you will ever think she's ready?"

Bree looked at Knox. She knew he was right. She'd had Ally all to herself almost from the time she was born. She knew it was selfish to want to hold on to her this way. And Knox wasn't asking for her to give Ally to him. He was just asking for her to share her niece with him. And he was right; she'd never think Ally was ready for this news. How could you prepare a little girl for something like this?

"I'm Ally's father, Bree. The longer we keep this from her, the worse it feels. She has the right to know."

"But what if she isn't ready? How do we tell her she had a daddy all this time and I didn't tell her about him?" Bree felt the tears begin to flow, but there was nothing she could do about it. "What if she hates me for keeping you from her? She's too young to understand that her mother had reasons that she thought Ally shouldn't know you.

"And what about the promise I made to my sister? I've already broke that once. I feel like I've let everyone down." Bree felt Knox's arms come around her. Laying her head on his shoulder, she spilled her last secret. "What if she grows up and realizes how much of this was because of my promise to her mother and how much of this was because I wanted to keep her all to myself?"

"It's going to be okay. We'll talk it out among the three of us. I'm not saying it's going to be easy. There's a lot that we need to figure out together. But we need to move forward, Bree." Knox moved away from her then and tipped her face up to his. "Ally loves you. Nothing that happens after this will ever change that."

Knox bent down toward her, his lips just grazing hers when a voice came from behind them. "Have the two of you forgotten that we have patients in the office? If you're going to be doing all this lovey-dovey stuff, you need to at least shut the door."

"I thought..." Knox began.

"We didn't mean to..." Bree said, then stopped when she saw the amused look on Lucretia's face. "Can you let my patient know that I'll be right there?"

"I can, but there's someone else you need to see first. That little girl, Megan. The one that those horrible human traffickers took. She's here with her mother."

Both Bree and Knox followed Lucretia out of the room to where a young girl who barely resembled the Megan they had met sat in the waiting room. There was no trace of makeup on the young girl's face and her hair had not only been washed, but had also been cut into a neat shoulder-length bob. Her clothes were clean and she looked like she'd gained some weight. Bree was sure that there would always be trauma left from her experience, but it was easy to see that she was on a good track for recovery. Beside her sat a woman not that much older than Bree. She was pretty like her daughter, but Bree recognized the fatigue and stress in the woman's eyes. The woman had gone through hell while searching for her daughter.

"We wanted to bring you these," the woman said, standing when they entered the room. "Megan helped make them. She wanted to thank you and the police officers for everything you did for her."

"Thank you. We were glad that we could help." Bree knew that they'd only offered the girl food and a phone call, but it was those two things that had gotten the girl off the streets and back with her mother. What wrong turn Megan and her mother had made didn't matter now. All that was important right now was that they were back together. With help, hopefully the two of them would work things out and be okay.

While Knox and Megan's mother talked, Bree went to look for her own little girl. Seeing the teenager who had once been in so much danger made it seem all the more important that she hold Ally close. She knew that Knox wasn't going to take Ally and run away with her. She knew Knox would never endanger his daughter in any way. But after all the years of providing for Ally all by herself, it was hard for her to think of giving some of that control up to Knox.

When Bree found the reception office empty, she began to go through the exam rooms. When she got to the one that held her patient, the only one left in the office, she listened at the door, thinking Ally had probably gone in to talk to the woman while she waited, even though she'd been warned to stay out of the occupied rooms. But when she entered, she found that her patient was there alone. Excusing herself again, with the promise that she'd return as soon as possible, Bree went to the bathroom at the end of the hall. There were only so many places where Ally could be in the small offices. Knocking on the bathroom door, then opening it to find it empty, the panic that had begun to rise inside her burst out. "Ally? Ally? Where are you?"

Bree rushed back through each room, calling out for her little girl. When Knox met her in the hallway, she was shaking so badly that she could barely get the words out of her mouth. She had experienced this once when she and a three-year-old Ally had been shopping and the toddler had decided to hide in a clothes rack where Bree couldn't see her. There was no way to describe the fear you felt when your child was suddenly gone.

"What's wrong? Where's Ally?" Knox asked, taking Bree's shoulders and steadying her.

"She's gone. Ally is gone."

Bree's words made no sense to him. His daughter had been there just minutes before, playing with her Barbie dolls on the floor by Lucretia's chair. Leaving Bree, he rushed to the receptionist office to see the dolls lying on the floor. He started back toward the other rooms when Bree stopped him. "I've already looked everywhere. She's not there."

"What's happened?" Lucretia said, coming from the waiting room where she had gone to show Megan and her mother out.

"I can't find Ally. Was she with you?" Bree asked.

But Knox could see by the shock in Lucretia's face that she didn't know where the little girl was. "I'll call the security guard and have him start looking for her."

Knox took Bree's hand as Lucretia rushed to the office phone. "We'll start on this floor and work our way down."

"But what if she went outside? Oh, God. What if she was taken?" Bree pulled her phone out. "Lucretia, call 911. And call me or Knox if you find out anything."

Knox led Bree into the hallway, looking both ways, but seeing nothing. "She couldn't have gone very far."

"I don't understand why she would have left the office at all. We talked about this. She knows not to go anywhere without an adult. I don't even let her be outside our house without me with her."

Knox tried to think of some reason Ally would have left the office and where she would have gone. "Maybe she's just playing with us. Kids don't understand that sometimes playing like that can be dangerous."

He stopped at the first office they came to and looked

around the room. "I'm sorry to interrupt, but have you seen a little girl? A blonde? Green eyes?"

"She was wearing jean shorts and a pink-and-purple plaid shirt," Bree said, her body trembling when she joined him in the doorway.

When the woman in the office shook her head, they moved on. They had visited each office on the floor, looking closely at the children in the waiting room at the county pediatric clinic. But Ally wasn't there.

They had started down the stairs when Bree's phone rang. "Hello? Ally?"

Knox tried to listen to the person on the other line but they spoke too quietly. When Bree hung up and her legs went out on her, Knox caught her and lowered her to the nearest step. Her face was paler than usual and then she began to cry.

"What is it?" Knox asked, holding Bree by the shoulders. "Tell me."

Knox had been through many tragedies in his life. He'd lost friends and loved ones. He'd held babies that had never taken a breath. He'd held the lives of patients and their babies in his hands during emergency surgeries. He'd even been in danger himself at times when he found himself up on a mountain, driving around their hairpin turns in snowstorms or torrential rains. Nothing scared him like the look in Bree's face at that moment.

"They found her. She's in the security office downstairs," Bree said, her voice shaking with each word.

Then she lost it, there on the steps of that old, rundown county building. All Knox could do was hold on to her as the tears began to run down his face, too.

They made it to the security office as soon as they got themselves together. But when they walked in, Knox was surprised to find a solemn Ally that made no move to run to them.

"Oh, Ally, you scared me so much," Bree said, not seeming to notice that the little girl didn't hug her back. "Why did you leave the office? You know that you can't go anywhere without an adult with you."

"I don't want to talk to you," Ally said, pulling away from her.

"What? What's wrong, sweetheart? Is this about the trip to the ranch? I told you that me and Dr. Knox needed to talk about that. Being mad about that isn't a reason to run away and scare us like that."

Knox could see that Bree's fear of losing Ally was beginning to dissolve. She had moved on to wanting answers and he had an idea what those answers would be. Bending down so that he was on his daughter's level, he met her eyes. "Ally, did you listen in on a conversation between me and your aunt?"

The girl only showed the slightest hint of guilt before she put her chin up in the air. "You said that you were my daddy and Aunt Bree doesn't want me to know."

Knox heard Bree catch her breath, but he didn't look up. "Me and your aunt were having a private conversation. If you heard us say something that you didn't understand or that made you angry, you should have let us know you were there. Running off wasn't the right thing to do. You scared us badly. If you ever hear something that scares you or that you don't understand, I want you to tell one of us so we can explain it to you."

He didn't want to scold his daughter. She'd heard something that she shouldn't have overheard and she was probably as much confused as she was scared. That was on him and Bree. But he also couldn't allow her to think that running away would be the answer when she was angry or scared.

Bree bent down and joined them. "I'm sorry that you overheard us. We were both trying to find a way to tell you, but I wanted you to have some time to get to know Dr.... I wanted you to get to know your daddy before we told you. I know you have a lot of questions and we're going to try to answer them the best we can."

Ally looked from him to Bree, then back to him. "Are you really my daddy?"

Knox looked his little girl in the eye. Green eyes, so unlike his own, but still there was something in the stubborn glint of them that reminded him of his mother. "Yes, Ally. I'm really your daddy."

CHAPTER TWELVE

WHILE BREE TALKED to the police officer and the Children's Services officer, Knox took Ally over to a corner where they could talk. "Do you have any questions for me while your aunt Bree is talking to the officers?"

"Did I get her in trouble?" Ally said, biting her lip in the same cute way Bree sometimes did.

"Your aunt can take care of this. Just like she's always taken care of you."

"Does your being my daddy mean that I won't live with her anymore?"

Right when Knox thought he was prepared for anything his daughter could ask, she surprised him. He'd thought she'd have questions about how he and her mother had met. How was it that he didn't know that she was his daughter? Questions that he'd have asked. Instead, she'd asked something that was much more simple. At least it should have been. "Me and your aunt are still trying to work out the details. How do you feel about it?"

He knew these were things that he and Bree should be discussing with her together, but the choice of time and place had been taken away from them when Ally had overheard them talking.

"Don't you like Aunt Bree?" Ally asked.

"Of course, I like your aunt a lot." He wasn't about to try to explain the crazy emotions Bree made him feel to his daughter. He was still trying to understand them himself.

"Do you want to kiss her?" his daughter asked. "My friend at school, Danny, says his parents kiss because they love each other."

Knox was going to have to find out who this Danny kid was and why he was talking to his daughter about kissing. He looked over to where Bree spoke with the officers. There was nothing he'd like more than to kiss away the worried look on her face right then. "Yes, I want to kiss her."

"Then why can't we all live together?" Ally asked, her face turned up to him.

How did he explain to her how complicated adult relationships were? But did it really have to be that complicated? Wasn't the simple truth that his feelings for Bree had grown into something much more than those he should have for his daughter's aunt or for the midwife he worked with? Hadn't his fascination with her freshness, her spirit, the way she stood up to him, started long before he even knew about his daughter? Hadn't he felt something forming between the two of them the day they'd delivered the baby at the clinic when she'd smiled at him and it had suddenly felt like the two of them were the only two people in the world, and he was okay with that?

And then there was the night they'd spent together.

He'd never felt so whole, so complete, as when he'd held Bree in his arms that night. It was like pieces of the puzzle that had been his life that he'd scattered recklessly had suddenly come together. He couldn't imagine his life now without his daughter. He didn't want to imagine his life without Bree beside him.

He looked down to see his daughter staring at him with such faith in her eyes. Such faith in him, trusting that he would make everything right, when all along it was Ally's innocent reasoning that pointed him toward what he had wanted since the day her aunt had accused him of having his own fan club. If he'd ever had a fan club, there was only one person he would want in it. And that was Bree.

Bree sat beside Knox as he parked his truck in front of his parents' house. Facing Gail and Charlie Collins today wasn't something that she wanted to do today, but she knew she would have to face them at some point.

"So Ms. Gail is really my grandmother?" Ally asked for the hundredth time since they'd left their house.

"She's my mother and that makes her your grandmother," Knox said once more, with a patience that he should have won an award for.

But then again, he wasn't about to face his parents while trying to explain why they had never been told about their granddaughter before now. Knox had given them the news over the phone and he said that they had taken the news well, that both of them were excited to learn that they had a grandchild even if they'd lost the first years of her life. Now it would be up to her to explain just how she had kept them from their only grandchild.

"It's going to be okay," Knox said, taking hold of her hand.

He'd been quiet most of the ride there, answering Ally's questions easily, but saying almost nothing besides that. He'd even seemed nervous when he'd arrived to pick them up. The kiss he'd given her when Ally had run to get her backpack had been little more than a peck between friends. He seemed to be somewhere else. And considering what they were about to do, she needed him to be there with her. "Are you sure they won't run me out of town the moment they see me?"

"I can almost guarantee you that by the time the day is over they will be the happiest people in the state of Tennessee," Knox said, though she noticed his eyes didn't meet hers.

Ally, tired of waiting for the adults, undid her seat belt and opened the truck door, hopping down and running toward the house before Bree could make a grab for her. By the time Bree and Knox made it to the door, Ally was already opening it and running in as if she owned the place.

"Ally, stop. You didn't even ring the bell," Bree called from behind her. The Collinses were going to think she'd raised their granddaughter as if she lived in a barn. Of course, their barn was actually nicer than the house Ally lived in.

"That's okay," an older man said as he came down

the stairs. With hints of gray shooting through the same light brown hair that matched his son's, Charlie Collins had aged well. His skin was tanned and a little weather beaten, but as he walked toward them, she could see that he still had that swagger that had sent screaming women falling out into the aisles when he'd performed. His eyes were the same light gray as his son's, too. And right then he only had eyes for one person.

Ally stood staring up at him, her eyes studying him. "Dr. Knox, he's my daddy, he says that you are my grandpa. Are you okay if I call you grandpa or will it make you feel old? My friend Josie says that she doesn't call her grandmother Grannie because her grandmother says it makes her feel old. I can call you something else if you'd like me to."

Charlie Collins looked down at the little girl before he broke out in laughter as loud as if he had a mic hidden in the beard running down his chin. "I think I'd like to be called Grandpa. And what shall I call you?"

"My name is Ally. Ally Rogers. And this is my aunt Bree. You can call her Bree, though, because you're an adult."

"It's nice to meet you, Bree," Charlie said, nothing but politeness in his tone.

"It's nice to meet you, Mr. Collins."

"There she is," Gail Collins said, coming down the stairway behind her husband. "How are you doing today, Ally?"

Ally ran up the stairs and met Gail. "I'm fine. You're my grandma."

"So I've been told," the older woman said, taking Ally's hand as she continued down to where Bree waited. "Charlie, why don't you take Ally down to the basement to see the playroom? If I remember correctly, our granddaughter likes to play those video games you have down there."

"Can I go?" Ally asked Bree. When Bree nodded, Ally let go of her grandmother's hand and grabbed hold of Charlie's.

"I thought I'd saddle up a couple of horses for me and Bree. I'll be right back," Knox said, giving Bree an encouraging smile before heading back out the front door.

Bree watched him retreat, leaving her alone to face his mother. "I guess I owe you an explanation about why I didn't tell you about Ally when we were here."

"Let's sit down a moment," Gail said, moving over to where four leather chairs faced a large fireplace. "Knox has explained most of everything, at least everything he knows."

"I've told him everything that I know myself. I wasn't in Brittany's life at the time so I can only say I think she had reasons for the way she handled the pregnancy. Maybe if she hadn't been killed, she would have changed her mind. I don't know."

"If it's not too painful, do you mind me asking why you and Brittany weren't communicating? Knox said you didn't even know she was pregnant until after Ally was born."

"When I look back, it was stubbornness on both of our parts. Brittany wanted a life in country music. I wanted to go to college and then medical school. She felt that my refusing to perform with her had ruined her chances of that life. I didn't think so. I still don't. Don't get me wrong, she had a beautiful voice, but there are a lot of beautiful voices in Nashville."

"I'm glad you got to go into medicine, but midwifery? That wasn't in your plan, was it? But then I'm sure raising Ally wasn't in your plan, either. You had to have considered telling Knox about her at some point. You had to know that you could have gone on to medical school if he'd taken Ally."

Knox taking Ally from her had never crossed her mind. She'd done her best to honor her sister's promise, until she'd had proof for herself that her sister was wrong. "Ally's not just my niece, Mrs. Collins. She's my child in every way. I never thought of giving her up to anyone. I did what was asked of me by my sister. Neither of us knew that within a few hours she would be dead."

"I'm sorry. I don't want to upset you. I have no doubt you did what you thought was best for Ally. I could see the love you two share when Knox first brought the two of you to the ranch. I thought then that maybe Knox had finally found someone that he could have a steady relationship with. Then I find out that it wasn't you that he was interested in, it was Ally. It's taking me a few moments to believe that."

They both stood when Knox came into the room. "Ready?"

"Yes, but is it okay if Ally stays here?" Bree asked Knox's mother. Their whole conversation was confusing to her. She couldn't tell if the woman was angry at her or if she truly was trying to figure out how all of this had taken place. And Bree had to admit, her saying that Knox was only interested in Ally had hurt, even if Knox's mother hadn't meant for it to.

"Of course. This is her home now as much as it is Knox's. Besides, I have an interior decorator arriving soon to help us make one of the rooms here just for Ally."

Not knowing what to say to that, Bree followed Knox outside. He helped her mount a sweet, gentle mare before he climbed up on his own horse. "I haven't been on a horse in a while. When I was young, me and Brittany took lessons. It's one of the few things I regret not being able to give Ally."

"I don't think you need to worry about that now. We'll make sure she gets lessons," Knox said, leading the way across a field that ran behind the house.

"Are you okay?" Bree asked. "You've been quiet all day."

"I'm fine," he said. "There's a path I want to take you up to on that hill. Then we need to talk."

His words had an ominous tone to them. What had happened since the two of them had talked last that would have made him change so much? And what had he meant when he said that *we* would make sure that Ally had riding lessons? Did he mean the two of them, together? Or was he talking about him and his parents? Anytime Knox had brought up helping Bree pay for Ally's support, she'd shut him down. She knew that at some point she'd have to accept that Knox had the right and the responsibility to help with Ally's expenses, but it was hard to take money from someone when she'd worked so hard to support the two of them on her own.

And what had his mother meant by having a room decorated for Ally? Did she think that Ally would be moving in here? Was that what Knox wanted?

And then there was the comment of his mother's about Knox being just interested in his daughter. Had he not told her that the two of them were involved? Or was that all in her own imagination? She knew that people had sex and then moved on; wasn't that what her own sister and Knox had done?

Was that it? Had she been just as naive as her sister, thinking that she and Knox were building a relationship together?

By the time they got to the top of the hill, Bree was beginning to fall apart. Had she really fallen for a man so devious that he would use her to get his daughter?

That thought stopped her in her tracks. Or in her horse's tracks. No matter what she might think, she knew that Knox Collins didn't have a devious bone in his body. If he did plan to take his daughter away from her, which she had to admit was his right as Ally's father, he would never do it backhandedly. He'd tell her gently, letting her down as easy as possible.

Yeah, he'd do something like take her on a horse ride in the country.

"Stop!" The sound of her own voice startled her as it echoed into the hills.

"What's wrong? We're almost there," Knox said.

"If you're going to tell me that you're going to take

Ally away from me, I'd rather do it before we go any farther," Bree said.

Knox jumped down off his horse and came back to her. "What are you talking about?"

"I don't want you to try to sugarcoat this. Just tell me the truth. Are you going to take Ally to live with you?"

"Yes, I want Ally to live with me. That's something I wanted to talk to you about," Knox said, then reached up and pulled her out of the saddle and into his arms. "And before you start imagining the worst, though I have the feeling that you already have, maybe you should listen to me."

Bree pushed against him until he placed her down on her feet, then started up the path, leading her horse behind her. "How can I not imagine the worst when you've barely said ten words to me today and you have a mother who's right now making plans to decorate a room for Ally?"

"I haven't felt like talking because I've been trying to find a way to talk to you about this. But you've already jumped to the conclusion that I would just take the child that you have raised like a daughter away from you. Does that really sound like something I would do to you? Is that really what someone who loves you would do to you?"

Bree stopped, her horse bumping against her, making her lose her balance. Sitting there in the dirt, she looked up at Knox. 'You love me?"

"Yes, I love you. I was hoping that you loved me, too. I had this great speech I had been working on. A fancy one where after I've taken you to the top of this hill, I tell you about how all of this will be mine one day, but none of it would mean a thing if you weren't there beside me." Knox sat down beside her. "Stupid, huh?"

"Maybe a little bit. You know that I don't care about any of this stuff. I care about you and Ally. The two of you are all I need, too." Bree leaned against him then, putting her head against his shoulder. Leaning forward, she took his face in her hands and kissed him. "I love you, Knox Collins."

When they pulled apart, Knox stood and offered her a hand. "I might have brought a blanket and some wine in my saddlebags, if you want to climb up this hill with me."

Bree put out her hand, knowing that when she took his hand her whole life was about to change. "Knox Collins, nothing would make me happier than the two of us climbing this hill and every other one that life puts in front of us, together."

EPILOGUE

"IS THAT it?" Knox asked her for the third time. She'd told him when he rented the trailer that it wouldn't be big enough for everything she and Ally needed to take with them.

It had been three months since they'd told his parents that they were all moving in together. It had only been two weeks that Knox had gotten the call about a building he had been looking at to start a new clinic, one that both he and Bree could work at together now that she had passed her examinations and received all her certifications.

"Did you get Maggie's blanket?" Ally said, carrying her new puppy that her grandparents had insisted she needed if she was going to be moving away from her friends. They might just as well have bought their daughter a pony by the looks of the curly-haired dog's enormous paws.

"Her blanket and her bowls are in the back of the truck. Why don't you climb in and get her settled." Bree helped Ally up inside the truck then turned to the friends who had come to see them off.

"I had really hoped the two of you would settle down here in Nashville," Sky told her as they hugged.

"We'll be back next month for your and Jared's wedding," Bree said, wiping at her eyes.

"And then you'll be coming back for your own wedding this Christmas," Lori said as she shared a hug with the two of them.

Bree looked down at the diamond that glittered on her finger. It was a beautiful ring, but it was the question that Ally had asked when she and Knox had shown it to her little girl that had been the brightest moment of the night. "Because you are marrying my daddy, does that mean you will be my mommy now?" It had been a night of laughter and tears, and she would remember it always.

"You ready?" Knox asked, shaking Jared's hand before climbing into the truck. Bree turned back to look at the little house where she'd worked so hard on her own to make a home for her and Ally.

But now she wasn't alone. She and Ally had Knox. They'd gone from two to three, and they were even talking about adding a fourth one to their numbers, though they hadn't shared that with Ally yet.

Climbing into the truck, she looked over at the man she loved, the one she wanted to share all her new adventures with. "Yes, I'm definitely ready."

* * * * *

FAKE DATING THE VET

JULIETTE HYLAND

MILLS & BOON

For my spicy kitty, Groot.
Without his constant "snuggles" on top of my laptop,
this book might have been turned in on time!

CHAPTER ONE

THE PRISTINE WHITE paper with black and white flowers stood out on Dr. Violet Lockwood's desk. Fiona's wedding invitation had arrived almost five months ago. And she'd sent along her RSVP and plus-one four months ago.

It was the plus-one causing her issues now. Why hadn't she just marked that she would attend alone? Violet pinched her eyes closed and took a deep breath. She knew exactly why... because Thomas would be there.

With his new wife.

The one who looked just like her according to the texts she'd gotten when they started dating. His date was the woman he'd actually met at the altar.

If she'd RSVP'd honestly, she'd have had four months to get used to the stares she knew would come her way. Four months to practice her smile among the friend group she'd been so close to in college. Four months to find self-deprecating jokes about how the woman who'd craved a partner was stranded in perpetual singlehood in Maine.

Four months to ready her armor for Thomas's barbs.

Hell, she could have been truthful when Fiona asked her about her date a month ago—owned up to the lie no matter how embarrassing the whole thing was. She could even have lied, said that the relationship just hadn't worked out.

But no. Those were not the sensible paths she'd chosen.

Violet had bragged about how hot the mythical man was, how good he was in bed, how excited she was for everyone to meet him. All without ever giving away a name. A ploy Fiona had been too kind to call her bluff on.

Now she was two weeks away, with the plate of chicken she'd ordered for the imaginary date. She'd meant to call Fiona and tell her to cancel it weeks ago. Own up to her failure.

She could still make that call. At least that way the servers wouldn't ask if anyone was coming to the empty place beside her. Violet had used up every excuse in the book. Even now the invitation was on her desk so the excuse of getting home too late to call after working as the on-call emergency vet vanished.

That was her plan a week ago when she'd dumped it in her backpack and sworn for the twentieth time that today was the day she gathered her courage.

She looked at the clock, seven o'clock. She still had almost four hours left on her shift, but no patients at the moment.

Violet let out a breath, but she didn't reach for her phone. *Coward.*

"You stare any harder at that piece of paper, it might burst into flames. If it does, I want to video it. I mean how often does that happen?"

"Never, Beck. That *never* happens." Violet rolled her eyes at the vet tech who was hotter than any man had a right to be. And, at twenty-six, ten years her junior, Beck Forester was so not in her dating pool.

That didn't stop her subconscious from filling her dreams with illicit things.

The man was just over six foot, with broad shoulders and the ability to dead lift an injured 110-pound Great Dane. And yet somehow he managed to sneak up on everyone in the clinic where she was a staff veterinarian.

He also blew through his annual vacation as fast as he earned it, jetting to far-off places whenever the whim set in. Two months ago, his hike through part of the Appalachian Trail was interrupted by a far too close call with a cougar. The man had stories that could keep you entertained for days.

"Never is a long time. It *could* happen." He winked, then pointed to the invitation. "What has you so cross about a wedding invitation, Doc?"

What indeed?

She laid the invitation down. "Think every wedding invite looks the same so it's obvious to nosy vet techs what someone is looking at even without reading it?"

"Maybe." Beck shrugged, not a care in the world. In the nearly two years they'd worked together, she'd never seen the man worry. Never watched a frown cross his lips. No pinched eyebrows or terse words to indicate he was having a bad day.

Nope. Beck always had a smile and was ready for whatever adventure came his way that day. The man was the definition of go with the flow.

Once upon a time she'd been good at that, too. A chance to go to overseas for an agility competition—yes please! Girls' trip just because—of course.

That was a lifetime ago and a very different Violet.

"That invite has been on your desk all week, right by a notepad that says 'call Fiona.' I saw it when I was grabbing Maverick's file, and then again when I came looking for Jack's. Sooner or later Dr. Brown is going to have to drop the paper system. And then the supplier will go out of business as I think he may be keeping them in the black all on his own."

He was giving her an out. A way to discuss something else.

It was kind. And the topic of overflowing paper files was one every member of the office, except Dr. Brown, chatted about regularly—even though they all knew the answer.

The office would get a new system when Dr. Brown finally sold it. Probably to one of the corporate companies that came by every few months offering very generous buyouts. So far, Dr. Brown said he had no interest, but eventually the dollar signs would be enough.

Everyone had a price.

"I am a bridesmaid in a wedding in less than two weeks." Violet threw the invite on the desk. "I RSVP'd with a plus-one and never canceled the date. I hate the idea of going alone. Want to pretend to be my boyfriend for a weekend in Florida?"

"Oh, I am absolutely down for that. What part of Florida?" Beck looked seriously excited. For a moment she thought he might clap.

Violet opened her mouth but no words came out. She wasn't sure what was more shocking. That she'd made such an offer or that she ached to leap at the option too.

Beck jumping wasn't surprising at all. This was the kind of thing he lived for. He'd make the perfect date.

"The wedding is in Miami." Nope. Those were not the words that were supposed to come out. Shutting this down should be her goal. But Beck was hot. He would turn heads. But more importantly, he was kind.

If Thomas pulled anything, and knowing her ex he absolutely would, Beck would have her back. Fake date or not, on his arm this wedding had a chance to actually be fun.

"Cool. I have never been to Miami. How long have we been 'dating' for this ruse?" Beck made air quotes around the word *dating*.

"Beck." This was rapidly spinning out of control. He was

excited, and for the first time in months she wasn't dreading what should be a happy occasion.

"I can't ask you to do this." Though in her head she was already plotting how to get him on the plane with her. She had a ticket…but he would need one too.

And with only two weeks to go, ticket prices would be astronomical.

"You already did." Beck grinned showing off the deep dimples in both cheeks. Of course the Adonis had dual dimples. That was another thing her brain insisted on imputing into her dream life. "Now I just need the details."

This was fully out of control. As great as it would be to walk into the wedding on Beck's arm, she couldn't do this. Shouldn't do it. She didn't need a man. She was thirty-six. She was a veterinarian. Her life was boring but it was hers. Her terms. Period. "Beck—"

"Violet." He mimicked her tone as he interrupted her. "I have a ton of mileage points, so my ticket will be free. I assume you already have a hotel room. I'll go halfsy with you on it, if I can sleep on the pullout couch. Do I need my tux for this or will a suit work?"

He clapped. The hot, twenty-six-year-old Adonis actually clapped at the idea of attending a wedding with her. "Or is it a beach wedding and I get to wear a swimsuit? I draw the line at a nude wedding." Beck put his finger on his chin, closing his eyes. "I mean maybe for the experience I could go to a nude wedding…"

"No! No." Violet blinked as the wall of words and the image of a nude Beck on the beach gripped her brain. "No, it's black tie. Why do you have a tux?" Any question would work to try to get the spicy thoughts from her mind.

Beck chuckled as he moved; his tall frame sliding into the

tiny office chair with such ease. "For occasions like this." He held up a hand, clearly anticipating a sharp retort.

"I'm not joking. For occasions like this. I found one at a thrift store in Texas on a trip a few years ago. Got it for less than twenty dollars and had it tailored. Now, I have it for a wedding date in Miami. The world is full of opportunity if you are willing to jump at it."

Right. That had been her motto once, too. That Violet had traveled the world, jumped at anything that sounded like fun. Fallen in love fast—and been devastated by the results. Lost her entire life in the process.

She'd rebuilt, but she wasn't the same person. One did not get to go back to the person one was after coming home to find the place practically cleaned out—after getting stood up at the altar.

"So it's black tie. We leave next Friday?"

"Yeah, on the first flight out. The rehearsal dinner is at six. I have handled all my bridesmaid duties long distance. Luckily, Fiona is the exact opposite of a bridezilla." Surely she wasn't actually going to do this. It was too much.

"Beck—"

"You on this five-thirty flight out? A layover in DC and then onto Miami?"

"Yes, but…"

"Cool. Booked. No backing out now, Violet. My points are nonrefundable. But I will warn you I am not a morning person. There is a reason I work the late shift." He held up his phone and playfully raised his eyebrows.

"Considering we will basically go from our shift to the airport, I won't hold it against you." This was happening. Really happening.

A fake wedding date. This should be a new low. But the twinge of excitement in her belly refused to accept any shame.

"So, what roles are we playing? I assume this is to get back at an ex."

Beck rubbed his hands together, and she couldn't help but laugh. "Why are you so into this?"

"Come on, Violet. How often do you get to pretend to be dating someone? It's like our own television drama. I am not missing out on this. So again, who are impressing?"

"You will impress everyone who sees you." Violet put her hand over her mouth, heat flooding her cheeks as Beck leaned a little closer. Damn the man was hot. And he knew it.

He cocked his head, those dimples appearing as he stared at her.

"My ex-fiancé." Violet rolled her eyes. "He left me at the altar…via text. An hour before we were supposed to say I do. He and his new wife will be there. It's dumb, but I don't want to deal with questions and pitying looks."

"Why go at all? Surely your friend will understand."

"Because Fiona and I were college roommates. She was my maid of honor, she passed me tissue after tissue while I cried over the lout who didn't show. Unfortunately, her soon-to-be husband is stepbrothers with Thomas. The two of them aren't close, but he doesn't want to upset their father. The man is getting on in years."

Violet blew out a breath. "Besides, it will be fun to see my old girlfriends. I am the only one who left the area." Fled was the actual term, but she was already dumping too much info on him.

She'd sold her and Thomas's condo, a task made infinitely easier by the fact that the only thing he'd left her was the un-opened wedding gifts, her bed and clothes.

Thomas had even taken her grandmother's cross-stitched tablecloth. He'd played dumb when she'd asked for it back. He said he didn't have it. That Violet must have misplaced it. Like she'd lose the one family item she cared about.

His mother had posted a picture of it last Christmas that a mutual friend had liked so it made it across her social media. So Thomas had it—and was using it.

The ass.

With little to her name, she'd accepted the job from Dr. Brown and rebuilt her life in Bangor. On her terms. And she was not letting a man mess with her peace again.

"I guess not inviting your ex would make future family get-togethers awkward." Beck delivered the line without bothering to hide the fact he disagreed with the decision.

Neither Fiona nor her lovely fiancé, Patrick, were happy with Thomas's attendance, but it made Patrick's dad happy. Sometimes you did what you could for family.

"So, we have been dating at least six months? Or do we go for a year? We could be engaged. Oh, what if I am a billionaire tycoon? Secret prince of some foreign island?"

Violet laughed. The small chuckle broke free into a raucous giggle, and she hugged her belly.

Beck's chuckle mixed with hers. A deep baritone that made her toes curl. Dear God, the man was positively delicious.

"I think you, on your own, Beck, are more than enough to get the tongues wagging. Plus all of the stories of your trips will make for dinner conversation." Heat spread across her body, into places she didn't think it should, as she leaned closer to him.

"Great. Six-month relationship that we are just now taking public because of your less than grand dating history. But I made you put down the plus-one so I could prove I would still be there for the wedding." He raised his brows as he created the perfect story for why she hadn't included his name.

Fiona might even buy it.

"Thank you." She bit her lip as emotions crept up her chest. This was the nicest thing anyone had ever done for her.

"Any time, Vi."

Vi. Only he shortened her name. It was something he'd done once about a year after he'd started at the clinic. The receptionist, Lacey, had quickly corrected him. No one called her anything but Violet, or Dr. Lockwood.

Her mother had hated nicknames and refused to call her anything but her full name. Control was her mother's coping mechanism in the world. Its impact on others was never her concern.

She'd gone by Vi in college—until she met Thomas.

Thomas had made a face the first time he heard it used. He said she was as delicate as a flower; one did not cut a flower short. By the end of their relationship, his focus on her beauty irked her, but in that moment, she'd thought he meant well.

Professionally she'd chosen the full name. Something she sometimes regretted.

Hearing Vi from Beck's lips always brought out a grin. Which was why she never asked him to stop and why she suspected he kept doing it.

"So, do we pass the slow evening talking about the wedding, or backstory, or gossip from your college years to make sure we seem like a long-term couple?"

"Uh." Right, there was more to this than just showing up on a hot guy's arm.

The front doorbell chimed and Violet held up her hands. "None of the above it seems. You jinxed us."

* * *

There was no way for Beck to kick himself without Vi notic-
ing. He'd been an emergency vet tech for nearly three years
now, two in this clinic. He knew better than to mention the
words *slow*, *quiet*, *tame*, *easy*. It was like asking for a rushed
case.

And he'd finally gotten an invitation to see her outside
the office. Playing her fake boyfriend would be the easiest
game he'd ever had. The woman was brilliant. Funny. And
drop-dead gorgeous. She must have men, and women, bang-
ing down her door to get a date but she refused to answer
the knock.

He'd had a crush on her since the second night they'd
worked together. A giant Great Dane had come in after eating one of his little human's socks, a surprisingly common
occurrence. The mom was panicking because she'd forgotten to pick up the toddler's sock. The toddler was in tears because puppy was sick. The dad was worried about everyone
and the vet bill.

Vi had sat on the floor, rubbing the giant dog's head while
she outlined all the options. When the father quietly explained
that they didn't have money if emergency surgery was needed,
she'd told him, without judgment, that most of the time they
could use other options.

The father had returned two days later—alone—tears
streaming down his face because the dog was worse. He'd
come to request euthanasia. Violet had explained that a donor
had stopped in to pay for care for any family that couldn't
afford it.

The relief on the patient's face as he took his sleepy dog
back home following surgery was seared in Beck's mind. As
was the knowledge that there'd been no outside donor. Vi had

done the surgery for free and taken the hit on the cost from her paycheck.

It was the first time he'd seen her act as the "mystery donor" but not the last.

Stepping into the reception area he was stunned to see Maria Miller and her border collie, Baby.

"Beck." Maria was on her feet, stress etched into the corners of her eyes.

"What is going on with Baby?" The border collie was basically Maria's child. The four-year-old pup was a champion agility dog. In fact, Baby was supposed to compete tomorrow at their local club. Though compete was little bit of an overstatement for tomorrow.

The gym hosted the monthly competition for fun, and more than one person came just for the potluck after.

"We were doing one more prep run; you know she loves them." Maria wiped a tear from her eye.

He could already see the blame taking over. "I know. This isn't your fault."

Baby, like most border collies, was highly driven. A breed bred to work, she was constantly on the go. He had his own border collie mix, Toaster. No matter how late he got home, he and Toaster would go through the agility course he'd set up in the back of the cottage he'd inherited from his parents.

"She let out a yelp as she ran down the A-frame. She tried to keep going." Maria buried her head in Baby's fur and let out a sob.

"The good news is she is walking. Let's get her into a room so Dr. Lockwood can take a look at her." Maria stood, holding on to Baby's leash, and followed Beck into the exam room.

He took Baby's vitals, then offered Maria a smile. "Baby is our only patient right now, so Dr. Lockwood should be in quickly." In the ER, patient arrival time didn't matter. It was worst-case scenario first.

He stepped out and found Violet waiting right by the door. Beck gave her the details quickly. She nodded, made a soft sound, then headed into the room. He followed.

"Did you run down the A-frame poorly, Ms. Baby?" Violet ran her fingers over the dog's head, scratching behind both ears. It was a nice petting for the dog, but he could see her monitoring Baby's tail.

It gave a few wags, but they were half-hearted at best. He'd interacted with Baby a lot while training Toaster. The dog was focused, but always wagging her tail.

"Which leg came up lame, Maria?" Violet looked at the woman.

She wiped a tear from her eye, then pointed to her back left leg. "It doesn't bother her when I touch it. And she puts weight on it. But she pulls it up anytime she picks up speed."

Sliding around the table, Violet reached for the knee and moved it slowly. "It's an ACL tear." Violet set the leg back down. "I can feel the instability in the joint when I move it.

"She probably tore it coming off the A-frame. The initial pain was what caused her yelp. Luckily, it isn't overly painful now. It's sore, and if she moves wrong, she will feel the instability and some pain. I am going to prescribe pain meds. Then have our evening receptionist schedule a nonemergency surgery time for Ms. Baby." Violet snuggled her face close to the dog. "We'll get you feeling better in no time."

"Yes—" Maria shook her head "—but that means we are out for the season. You and Toaster are the alternates for the intermediate team. Looks like you're up, assuming you don't have any fancy trips planned."

"A weekend trip to Miami, but otherwise I am free until regionals. Toaster and I can step in." Nancy had wanted him on the intermediate team to begin with. But Beck hadn't wanted to commit. He'd taken the role as alternate and would keep the promise to the team. But he hated the reason he and Toaster were stepping in.

Maria took a deep breath. "I'll let the Nancy know."

"I'll handle it." Beck rubbed Baby's head." You focus on your girl. She is your priority."

"Tell that to Nancy." Maria rolled her eyes.

The agility gym owner, Nancy, was the definition of high stress. The woman was bent on winning. The only problem was the other members of the gym cared about their dogs' health and happiness, not ribbons and trophies.

The intermediate team competed in regionals, but they'd never placed. Something only Nancy ever complained about.

Maria rubbed Baby's head. "Let's get you home, sweet girl." She waited for Beck to lift Baby off the exam table, then led Baby out of the room.

"Toaster ready for a competition?" Violet asked as soon as the door closed.

"Yes. She loves the course. You should come." He held up his hand before she could offer the polite "no thanks" she'd given every other time he'd suggested she come to agility training.

The whole gym had been thrilled when Dr. Violet Lockwood moved to Maine. She'd started training agility dogs as a child, been a champion as a teen and one of the most sought-after coaches in South Florida.

Endorsements, coaching fees and a bestselling, at least in the agility circuit, book were how she'd paid her veterinarian school tuition. Then she'd just quit.

No reason given on the team social media channel she'd

once made daily appearances on. Just a brief note to mention she'd parted ways with the South Beach Agility Training Group.

"We need to get to know each other a little better, if we are going to make your ex jealous." Beck was looking forward to learning more about the vet he spent so much time with but barely knew.

"I don't want to make him jealous. I just want to quiet any questions about my personal life." Violet crossed her arms, her chin rising just a little.

Damn she was fine.

"All right. That is your goal. *My* goal is to make him jealous." Beck pushed his hands into his scrub pockets.

"You have no reason to want to do that."

"He hurt you." Violet was one of the kindest people he'd ever met. And even if she wasn't, who texted...texted...their fiancée that it was over? An hour before they were supposed to get married.

That level of low deserved humbling. Period.

Rose crept up her cheeks as she broke eye contact. "Thank you."

His throat tightened as he stared at her. He coughed, trying to clear away the need rising around him. "Anyway, we need to look like a longtime couple to stave off the questions. I need to be at the event tomorrow evening, and we fly out in less than two weeks. The ruse needs to be perfect."

She bit her lip but then nodded. "I'll be there."

There was no way to stop the smile he felt creeping along his face. "It's a date."

"A fake date." Violet pointed a finger at him.

"A fake date," he conceded.

CHAPTER TWO

VIOLET RUBBED HER DOG, Bear's, head as she led him out of her car. The bully mix was around three. He'd been scrawny and missing most of his hair when she'd picked him at the shelter.

The all-white dog loved wearing sweaters, and Fiona had joked that Bear was Violet's dress-up doll the first time she sent his pictures to her. He was currently wearing a red shirt that said Stealing Hearts and Blasting Farts. It was the truest description of her big guy.

"You ready for tonight?" She looked at the training facility hosting this evening's team agility competition. It was tiny. Not even a third the size of the gym she and Thomas had owned in Miami. It had a homier look though.

Their third business partner, Mack, the one still on the title, had wanted everything sterile. Or as sterile as possible with dogs running around. Most agility dogs were family pets who loved to run courses. Their "trainers" were pet parents who wanted to engage extroverted dogs, find an outlet for animals that without a purpose would become destructive.

But at the highest level of the sport there were endorsements and cash prizes. It was a good living, if you could get there. And she had. With Thomas. They'd been sought after trainers; three of the dogs she'd trained had won national championships. Beating her ex's dog.

Thomas hadn't taken those wins well. And the gym hadn't won a national championship since she left.

Wins weren't what most people competed for. And it wasn't what most at the Happy Feet Dog Gym were after.

Beck had promised her that tonight they were only competing for a beat-up trophy that said Happy Retirement. It was an inside joke so old no one remembered how it had started. But the trophy was part of the gym's lore now, so it stayed.

"Vi!"

Her blood heated as she turned to wave to Beck and Toaster. The blue-eyed border collie was Beck's pride and joy. Bear started wagging his tail. Toaster was Bear's favorite at the dog park. Though he mistakenly believed he could keep up with the blue-eyed border collie as she raced around the dog park.

Bear always collapsed as soon as she put him in the back of the car. He wiggled his butt as Toaster stepped forward.

"Toaster is very excited to see you too, Bear." Beck rubbed Toaster's head and smiled at her.

He was in blue jeans that hugged his hips just right and blue T-shirt accenting the muscles on his arms. Her mouth watered as he rubbed Bear's head. If she hadn't sworn off relationships, she'd ask him out for real. A hot man who loved dogs was her kryptonite.

He probably kissed like a dream too. Slow, soft, then hard… Heat was pulsing in her cheeks. And other places.

Standing, he turned all his attention to her. "Can I kiss you?"

Her mouth fell open. Was her mind manifesting what she'd just imagined?

"Kiss your cheek, I mean." Beck cleared his throat and glanced away for a minute.

"My cheek?" Disappointment threatened to swallow her. This was no manifestation.

"We need to keep up appearances at the wedding. Pretending to be a happy couple now is probably good so awkward moments don't happen in Miami."

Awkward moments like this.

"Right." That made sense. Perfect sense. "Of course you can." She leaned forward a little, hoping the disappointment creeping along her spine would find its way out of her body.

The people in the gym knew them—or at least knew Beck. Knew he wasn't dating the ER veterinarian who went to work, home and the dog park. Violet was the definition of boring. She even had groceries delivered, now.

This hadn't been her plan. She and Thomas had traveled regularly on the training circuit. She'd even traveled overseas for several international competitions. Now though, her life was filled with work and nights in. She liked it—it would be nice if someone she cared about was beside her on the couch. But if Thomas had taught her anything, it was to not cede her peace to anyone.

Beck's lips were soft against her cheek. The touch gone too fast, but not quick enough for her body not to react.

She ran a hand down her neck, heat coating her fingertips as she tried to regain some composure. It was ridiculous to find such a quick moment so enticing. The man was playing her boyfriend, but that did not require her to act as though his touch lit a flame in her chest…and lower.

Beck wrapped an arm around her waist, but it felt more than a little off, as their dogs continued to jump and play together. "They look like they have been spending a lot of time together."

And we look awkward as hell.

She didn't voice that. She'd offered him the role of pretend boyfriend. Maybe Violet hadn't expected him to accept, but he had. Acting uncomfortable together wasn't going to achieve the goal she wanted.

In fact, it would stir up more questions. She'd started this adventure. She needed to see it through. Besides, a few weeks where she could touch Beck would hardly be a hardship.

"Can I kiss you?" She looked up at him.

He nodded, and she looked at him, drinking in the dimples on either side.

"Do I have something on my face?" Beck raised his left eyebrow.

"Just trying to decide which dimple to kiss." It was a silly statement but the truth.

"Personally, I suggest planting one on each, then deciding which is best." He leaned his left side forward, took her kiss, then turned the cheek and accepted one on his right. "So, which is the winning side?"

"Your left."

He made a tsking noise. "I always thought it was my right. Guess I've been posing in pictures on my bad side."

"You should rectify that." She hit his hip with hers, then pointed at the building. "Toaster needs to be warming up."

"Playing with Bear in the parking lot doesn't count?" There was that eyebrow raise again. Why did that motion make him look so dang cute?

"No. Do you usually have her jog around the perimeter, or up and down an A-frame a few times before starting her routine?" The words felt a little foreign. For years she'd spoken "agility" as a second language. A fluent recitation of workouts, routines, dog breeds and expectation management to unrealistic clients.

His deep chuckle stopped her in her tracks. "I don't have a standard routine. I am not sure any of us besides Nancy do. We compete in regionals because it is a fun trip out of state. And these Tuesday night competitions are less about competition and more about the potluck after."

"Potluck?" No one had told her about a potluck.

"No worries, I made a vat of chili." Beck squeezed her side.

"A vat?"

"Yes. It means large pot." He chuckled as she knocked her hip, a little harder than last time, against his. "The point is, I made a huge thing of chili that I dropped off a little while ago and picked up a thing of your favorite cookies at the store and brought them under your name. I wasn't risking letting you back out of coming tonight."

"How do you know my favorite cookie?" Violet let him open the door. She made Bear sit, waiting until the bully mix settled enough to follow the command, gave him a praise, then a hand command to walk through the door.

Beck did the same with Toaster, who obediently followed the command immediately.

"See how easy she makes it look?" Violet pointed to Toaster, who now seemed 100-percent focused on the training environment. Border collies were lovely pups, but the breed was bred to work. She always advised first-time dog owners to choose a less energetic breed to learn the ropes of dog ownership.

"Bear follows commands. He just takes a minute to think it over." Beck ran his hand along Bear's head, scratching behind her ears.

"Uh-huh." Violet gave Bear a playful scolding look, then turned her attention back to Beck. It was true though. Bear was very well-behaved. "You didn't answer. How do you know my favorite cookie?"

"You hide a box of chocolate-dipped shortbread cookies above your desk in the same cabinet where the extra-small and extra-large gloves are stored. Not the best hiding place. We all know they are there."

"I'm not hiding them from you guys. I'm hiding them from me." She let out a huff. She'd actually forgotten that was where she'd stored them a month and half ago. She'd torn out the bottom drawer of her desk certain she'd eaten them in the fog after a difficult ER patient.

She'd dated Thomas for two years, been engaged for two more and the man had insisted that her favorite cake was red velvet whenever anyone asked. Red velvet was a fine cake but the answer today was the same as it had been then—devil's food cake. She doubted her ex-fiancé paid any attention to the fancy cookies she purchased once a month, then hoarded for tough days to add a ray of sunlight.

And yet, Beck had noticed. Noticed and made sure there was a pack here tonight with her name on them.

"Thank you."

"No problem." He raised a hand, then pointed to the A-frame. "Vi says you need to warm up, and she is the expert. So let's go, girl." He offered Violet a small wave, then took Toaster out onto the field.

The man was sweet. And no one was ever going to say that watching him walk away in jeans hugging his perfect ass was a hardship.

Beck ran Toaster through her paces. Careful not to look over at Violet too often. The woman was like a magnet. The entire gym seemed to have found its way into her perimeter.

The expert they'd sought for years was finally here. From this vantage point it seemed like she was enjoying herself. He didn't want to hover. Vi could take care of herself, but as Nancy Perkins strode toward the vet, he motioned for Toaster to follow him.

Nancy was the gym's agility club president. The only one whose dog competed in competitions outside of regionals, and occasionally medaled. Never won, though. A complaint that was never far from Nancy's lips.

She'd not been quiet about her frustrations at Vi's continued refusal to join the gym. Even when everyone pointed out that Violet's schedule at the ER clinic made it difficult to be here when the gym was open and that her responses were always courteous. She'd written the book on the sport, literally, with what he now suspected was the ex-fiancé.

Stepping away from something was okay. As was rejoining…if you felt like it.

"Dr. Lockwood, good of you to *finally* join us."

Beck got to Violet's side just as Nancy let out the passive aggressive greeting.

"What finally brings you into our humble midst?" If Nancy was trying to win over the agility coach that had led multiple teams to international championships, this was the least likely way to accomplish it.

"I heard there was a big vat of delicious chili here." Violet met his gaze, her bright jeweled eyes glittering with her *What the f...* look he sometimes saw when pet parents made choice for their living breathing family member that made no sense.

"I don't know about delicious." He winked and slipped onto the bench next to her, wrapping an arm around her waist. They were playing pretend boyfriend and girlfriend, so the motion made sense. But he'd pulled her close because he didn't like the tone Nancy was taking.

Nancy's gaze slipped to his hand before she smiled. "So you're helping Toaster tonight?"

"I'm just here for the chili. And to root for my..." Her voice faltered as she looked away. "Root Beck on." Vi cleared her throat, then ran a hand over his knee.

His body flooded with need at the simple touch. "Why don't you come with me onto the course with Toaster? She needs to warm up more."

He stood, and Violet followed.

"Think Bear wants to come too?"

"You know he is too lazy for it." Vi wrapped her arm around his waist, squeezing him before letting go. The ghost of her touch clung to him.

Getting touched by Violet Lockwood over the next few weeks was not going to be a hardship.

"He likes the A-frame at the dog park." He couldn't help the chuckle that followed the phrase.

Vi playfully rolled her eyes to the ceiling. What Bear liked was barking at the dogs that ran up the A-frame, then running around it before lying under the shade. Bear had energy... when Bear wanted.

Otherwise he was perfectly content to lie around all day. Toaster was the exact opposite!

"All right, why don't you send her through the whole course." Vi gestured to the course, then made a hand sign to Bear. The sweet pittie sat, then lay down, putting his head on his front paws and letting out a friendly bark at Toaster.

"Looks like you have a cheering section." Beck snapped his fingers three times and headed toward the starting area.

He usually ran Toaster through the course one full time before she actually ran the course, just for familiarization.

She took off through the weave polls, then headed onto the seesaw, before hitting top speed at the first tunnel. She jumped over the single jump, the double, then flew through the hanging tire. When she pulled up at the end, Violet clapped.

Violet walked over, and he saw several people looking their way. Probably wondering how he'd found a way to get the famously hermit-like veterinarian to train Toaster. No one had asked about them arriving together, but the gym's gossips would be talking soon.

Hopefully their short fake dalliance wouldn't cause any issues. That was a potential problem for future Beck—his favorite activity was putting off tough issues to his future self. His mother had always said not to put off hard things… Beck saw no reason to accept difficulties until you absolutely had too. After all, the worries might disappear all on their own.

He caught Nancy leaning on the wall, carefully trying to catch any advice Vi might give him. She was going to be disappointed. Toaster didn't need training. His girl was having a blast, and so was he.

Beck was never motivated by prizes. It was the experience he craved. His mother had gotten unexpectedly pregnant with him in her late forties. His father was in his late fifties. They'd been thrilled after trying to get pregnant for years and losing the few pregnancies they'd had.

His parents had loved him deeply, but anything that might be slightly dangerous was not something they signed him up for.

Soccer…knee and concussion issues.

Football…traumatic brain injuries.

Swim team…drowning from exhaustion.

Gymnastics…broken necks.

They'd cared for him so much, but it wasn't until after he moved out that he got to try new things. Beck was motivated by the adrenaline rush.

"She looks like she is having fun." Vi stepped next to him. "And you positively beam when you are running with her."

"It's fun. Didn't you enjoy it when you ran the gym in Miami?" It was the wrong question. The second it was out of his mouth, she frowned, looking over her shoulder.

"I thought I did." Violet let out a small sigh.

"Vi?"

"What time does the competition start? I am looking forward to your chili." The words were clipped. She was not going to discuss Miami. Even though they were headed there soon.

Into the heart of a past she clearly didn't want to step into.

Reaching for her hand, he pulled her palm into his. She squeezed it but didn't drop the connection. So he took it a step closer and pulled her to him, wrapping his arms around her.

She leaned her head against his shoulder as he hugged her. He held her, looking at the clock. He'd read that twenty-second hugs were ideal to lower cortisol—the stress hormone.

After about fifteen seconds she let out a long sigh, but he didn't let go. Finally, she took a deep breath and stepped out of his embrace. "You didn't answer my question. What time does it start?"

"All right, everyone, let's get this started." Nancy clapped her hands and pointed to Bear. "If this one is participating, you need to join the gym. We can do paperwork after the competition."

"Just the cheering section." Violet snapped her fingers, and

Bear stood. "Good luck." She brushed her lips against his, the touch barely there, but for a split second everything and everyone around him disappeared.

Violet snapped her fingers again, and she and Bear started walking to the stands.

Callie, one of his friends, stepped up beside him. "You two are positively glowing. I even snapped a pic of it. So cute. I'll send it to you." She clapped her hands. "Guess now I know why you've turned down all my attempts to set you up."

Before he could find the words to explain why this was just fun, Callie was already dancing away. The woman was collectively known as the gym's worst matchmaker. Not a single pairing she'd orchestrated had ever worked out. But that didn't mean Callie was giving up.

She'd tried for the last year to find him a date. She was convinced he'd be happiest if he settled down. Maybe…one day.

He looked over at Violet. She raised a hand, giving a thumbs-up. He could feel the heat in his cheeks. The ghost of her lips against his.

Vi was kind. Great with animals. One of the smartest people he'd ever met. She was gorgeous, inside and out. But he wasn't looking for a partner.

Not now. Maybe not ever.

His parents had traveled the world. In fact, they'd met each other while hiking the Tour De Mont Blanc. They'd met in France and been head over heels in love by the time they'd crossed the Italian border.

His father had told him the story a million times. Stars in his eyes as he looked over at this mother. To hear his dad say it, they'd "gotten boring" after that. Bought a cottage in Bangor, Maine.

His father had taken a job at the University of Maine as a

professor of anthropology. His mother had worked as a civil engineer for the city of Bangor, creating a more sustainable city with winters that spent weeks well below freezing.

After they married the adventures were just retold stories in faded photographs and memories. That was not how he was going to live his life.

CHAPTER THREE

THE BACK DOOR CHIMED, and Violet didn't need to look over her shoulder to know that Beck had just walked into the clinic. The day techs finished an hour after Dr. Brown, and the other day shift veterinarians, so they could catch her up on any patients that would be staying with her until her shift ended at two.

Her cheeks heated as she listened to his footsteps come closer. She'd kissed him last night. Sort of. Her lips had brushed his just before he headed to the "competition."

Even now her fingers itched to trace her lips at the memory…something she'd done more than she wanted to remember last night.

"Hope you're hungry." Beck stepped to her side and dropped three glass bowls filled with chili. "I have lots of leftovers and no room left in my freezer, so I packed up dinner."

The top bowl had Lacey's name on it. That wasn't surprising; Beck seemed incapable of not considering others. Their receptionist worked the same late hours they did.

He bent his head, and for a moment she thought he was going to kiss her. She lifted her head, the motion automatic, and pursed her lips as he instead grabbed the bowl with Lacey's name and headed out.

Fire roasted her cheeks. Seriously. What was wrong with her? Yes, she'd kept herself walled off from relationships.

Walled off was an understatement. She'd accepted exactly two dates in the last year. Both epic failures.

But it wasn't like she was looking for anything special.

One failed engagement that resulted in so much fallout was more than enough to make sure you paid close attention to the person you were with. Sure she was lonely sometimes, or all the time. But loneliness was the price of keeping heartbreak at bay.

She'd missed every red flag with Thomas. And there had been *a lot*. That was a mistake she had no intention of making again.

Beck ignited a fire in her body despite all her intentions to keep her heart flame free. Probably because he was so hot. Physical attraction and years of self-induced celibacy were finally catching up to her.

"You feeling better about the wedding now?" Beck opened the door to the back room, placed his hand on the top of the door frame and leaned forward.

Damn. It took every ounce of willpower not to lick her lips at the sight.

Swallowing the lump of desire crawling up her throat, Violet looked at the notes from the day in front of her. "I've checked with the sitter for Bear. I know Julie is watching Toaster too. I hope she is ready to have our two plus her Pepper in the mix. They might have a wild weekend. My neighbor is going to water my plants. All I really have left is packing."

"That isn't what I meant."

She knew that. Knew he hadn't been checking to see if her bridesmaid dress was hung in the travel bag to avoid wrinkles or if the makeup she was using for the wedding was picked out and her town house ready to be empty for a few days.

"I don't know." Honesty. That was one way to handle this,

maybe even the best way. But she hated the shame hovering in the three words. It had been years. It shouldn't matter that Thomas was going to be there. Shouldn't matter that he'd found someone who looked just like her. Someone he'd showed up to marry.

"It's okay to be nervous." Beck didn't come closer, no hug today like there'd been yesterday. That was fine.

"I'm not nervous." She bit her lip. "I'm pissed." Violet blew out a breath. There was that honesty again.

"I mean…" Words failed to materialize.

"You mean?" Now Beck was moving toward her. His dark blue eyes trained on her.

Balling her hands, she tried to find words. What the hell, she'd uttered the truth out loud, may as well finish the conversation. "I lost so much when Thomas ended our relationship. He took all our stuff, pushed me out of our agility business. He even got Gran's holiday tablecloth. I mean why would even want my Gran's holiday cloth? That was just spite."

Violet felt like she was vibrating as words she hadn't let spill forth for years bubbled over. "He kept his head high while I cried over what I thought was a loving relationship only to realize I'd played the fool."

Besides losing the one family heirloom she cared about, that was the toughest part. Once he was gone, it was easy to see where all the cracks were. Easy to see why Fiona had checked not once, but three times in the month leading up to her wedding if she was really sure she wanted to do this.

At the time, Violet thought her friend was just worried she'd get cold feet. But nope.

She hadn't come from a loving home. Her parents stayed together for years out of spite. No one had wanted to lose face in the community for "breaking" their family. The lawyers had been hired right after Violet had graduated high school.

Even growing up watching an unhappy couple muddle through, she'd been so certain that she'd found true love.

Then he just walked away. If she'd had an inkling, any suspicion, maybe it wouldn't have been as hard.

But the truth was he'd always hated that she was too successful in their shared field to truly keep her under his thumb in the way that he'd wanted. No matter how small she learned to make herself it was never enough for his ego. But she understood it now. Had learned to look and evaluate every step. She was not losing herself again. Never again.

"I don't miss him, but man I wish I was the one going to this wedding with a new spouse on my arm, rather than dragging a fake date with me. No offense."

"None taken." Beck's arm wrapped around her shoulders, giving her a quick, tight, work-appropriate squeeze. "First of all, you're not dragging me. In fact, if I remember correctly, you tried very hard to take back an invitation that I jumped at."

She rolled her eyes.

"Careful. My mom always told me if I rolled my eyes too hard, they'd get stuck like that."

Beck only chuckled as she stuck her tongue out him.

"Second, no way for us to walk in married. The courthouse is already closed." He chuckled but never stopped watching her.

Her mouth was hanging open, even though she knew he'd offered the statement as a joke.

"But we can be dating. That way it isn't fake."

Violet's ears were ringing, and she wasn't sure he was making any sense. "Wha—"

"Vi, will you go on a date with me? A real one, besides to an agility gym?"

They'd acted the couple at the agility course last night. The simple kisses in the parking lot should have been the end of it. But she'd found herself reaching for his hand or enjoying it as his arm wrapped around her waist. Beck beside her while Nancy was a giant pill was nice, even when she'd failed to describe what they were to each other.

Last night was unexpected but comfortable. She did not want to tarnish that memory.

"I don't want a pity date, Beck. But I appreciate the offer."

His hands cupped her cheeks. "This is not a pity date. You are fantastic, Vi. Brilliant, funny, kind, pretty. I would *love* to take you out."

He'd called her pretty last. It was a silly thing to focus on, but everyone called her gorgeous. She knew she was conventionally attractive. Long wavy dark hair, a slim figure, high cheekbones. All things society deemed "special."

But those were also genetic things that she had no control over.

"You are very sweet."

Beck held up a hand. "I know a brush-off when I hear one, and I won't push, but we can go as people who are dating. It doesn't have to be exclusive. We can have a no strings attached fling that is just for fun. Your friends don't have to know it just started."

A fling. With Beck. Her toes curled in her sneakers as she tried to ignore the heat flashing through her body.

"Sounds pretty good to me." She popped a hand over her mouth as the words hung between them. Oh my. She'd meant to keep those words inside her head.

Both his dimples appeared as he raised his eyebrows again. "It *does* sound like a good idea."

Violet looked at Beck; he seemed genuinely interested. Dating a man ten years her junior was not something Vi ever planned to do. But returning to a wedding where her ex was wasn't on her bucket list either. They *were* going away for the weekend.

Once upon a time, Violet would have jumped at the chance to just have fun. To experience the moment.

Damn she missed that woman sometimes.

But that woman got hurt. That woman got her heart trampled. Still…

"Yes. I would very much enjoy going on a date with you. But—"

"Vi—"

"Hold on." She held up a hand. "We are coworkers. We should probably have some ground rules."

"Not a terrible idea." Beck reached for the hand she'd held up. He squeezed it quickly, then released it. "Rule one…"

Before he could finish that sentence, three quick buzzes rang over the speaker. That was the code for emergency.

She took off, knowing Beck was on her heels.

"My cat was hit by a car." A young man, no more than nineteen, was holding a small box.

"We'll do the best we can." Beck offered kind words, but she knew by the shift in his shoulders that the outcome was all but certain. He took the cat to the back to start vitals and triage.

"Lacey—"

"I'll get a room ready." A goodbye room. She didn't say those words, but the young man seemed to understand what was going on.

"Let's go over some options, while my vet tech looks at—"

"Minnow. His name is Minnow. Found him while I was fishing when I was fourteen. He was scrawny and in bad need of a bath, I didn't think my momma would let me keep him but…"

"Minnow is very lucky to have you." Violet took a deep breath. Tonight was going to be a rough shift—the life of an emergency vet.

Beck pulled up to Don's. The hideaway bar was relaxing, and on Sunday evenings Don hooked up a karaoke machine. It drew in an eclectic crowd.

It wasn't his typical first date hangout. But this wasn't a typical first date—and he was stunned Vi was even still willing to come out after yesterday's shift.

They'd lost the cat hit by the car, and two other emergencies had come in that were still very touch and go. It was one of those shifts that could make you question your choice in careers.

So he'd chosen Don's. Because it was tiny and people left you alone. And most importantly it was easy to lose any unhappy thoughts in the chaos that was people screeching out tunes. And given that Halloween wasn't all that far off, there was bound to be at least one silly rendition of "Monster Mash" every night.

"Beck." Vi held up a hand as she walked over from her bright yellow SUV. The car would never get lost in a crowded parking lot. Not that Bangor had too many of those.

She was dressed in jeans and a bright red sweater. "Let's get inside." Vi grinned as she hustled toward the door.

He followed. "You know most people wear coats once September is in the rearview mirror." October days were still decently mild, but the evenings were chilly and it was windy tonight.

Vi rubbed her hands up her arms as they moved toward the bar. "I hate bringing a coat into a restaurant or bar."

Beck put his arm around her shoulders to add some extra warmth to her. "There's the coat rack." He pointed to the corner where the hangers were already filling with brightly, and not so brightly, colored coats.

"My dad used to forget our coats when we were going out. Mostly to piss off my mom. She was very controlling and…" Vi shrugged. "I got used to just running into places when it was cold. They were always going to fight, but at least it wasn't going to be about my coat."

Vi chuckled as she leaned against the bar and ordered a beer. Beck didn't know what to say. That was clearly a story she'd told before, one she might even think was funny. But it was disturbing.

"You grew up in Maine?" He'd been born in Bangor. Graduated from Bangor High School, gone to vet tech school at the University of Maine Augusta campus…in Bangor and now lived in the home he'd been raised in. He traveled frequently. His passport was filling with stamps, and he'd visited thirty of the fifty US states already. But somehow, the home coated with happy memories with his parents was where he always came back to.

"No." Violet thanked the bartender as she held up her beer and headed for a booth on the back wall.

He grabbed his drink and followed.

Sliding into the booth, Vi took a deep sip of her drink, then let out a sigh. "I grew up in Kansas. So not as much snow as here, but the wind in the winter BITES. Nothing but flat land so no wind breaks. I moved to Florida for college, and to put more than a thousand miles between my parents and me."

Once more she'd stunned the words from him. His parents had protected him—a little too much. But he'd never wanted distance between them. Even now, he had several pictures of their adventures in his living room so he could feel close to them on the days when his soul ached that all he had left was their memory.

"All of that is information I don't normally share on a first date." She looked at her beer, spinning the bottle around by its neck. "But it's information Fiona would expect you to have."

"Right." Somehow the fact that he needed to pass the boy-friend test at least one of her friends would throw his way had slipped his mind.

"Do you have a coat in the car, at least?" This part of Maine was no stranger to poor weather even in October. People started making sure their trunks had coats, blankets and kitty litter you could put under your tires to create friction against ice if you slid off the road at the end of September.

"Of course." Vi's nose twitched and she pursed her lips. "It's nearly winter."

"Give me your keys." He held out his hand.

Vi kept spinning the beer bottle. "Why?"

"Because I am going to grab your coat. We'll hang it right by mine. So it's nice and warm when you go outside."

"Beck, it's fine."

"No." He shook his hand. "Your keys, Vi."

She rolled her eyes but fished them out of her jeans pocket. "It's not necessary."

Beck tilted his head. "I think we have very different ideas of necessary in this situation. I promise I won't let you for-get it."

Running outside, he grinned as he pulled open her SUV's door. She had two key chains hanging from a lanyard on her rear view mirror. One said, *Therapy isn't enough. I need to bite people.* The other was a coffee cup that read, *My blood type is coffee.*

The lanyard with the key chains fit the bright yellow car. He grabbed the coat off the passenger seat and headed back in. After hanging it on the hook next to his, he headed back to his date.

"If I forget my coat, I am never letting *you* forget it." She playfully wagged a finger at him, then looked up at the stage as the first karaoke performer started up.

He wasn't going to let her forget her coat. But there was a more important issue at hand now.

"We have to have a bet."

"A bet?"

There wasn't time for a long explanation. "When will some-one sing 'Monster Mash'? Three songs in? Five in? Last of the night? It's October, the holiday tune *will* come up."

Vi covered her mouth, but her eyes were bright with a smile. "'Monster Mash'?" She looked at the performer, flip-ping through the song book.

"I say it's between the fourth and eighth performance." Beck leaned a little closer, enjoying the happiness radiating from her.

"I say the last one, or the last one we are here for. I know we usually work the night shift, but closing the bar down on our night off is no guarantee."

"Fair." He'd spend as much time as she wanted at the bar. But he also understood the need to head home after decom-pressing.

The first song started, "Bohemian Rhapsody."

"That is ambitious!" Vi looked at the singer, then turned back to him. "What are we betting for? Usually that is decided before the bet is even outlined, but we had to rush tonight."

"Who kisses who first." Beck winked.

Kiss. Her mouth went dry. He wasn't talking about the soft, barely there kiss she'd given him the other night. No, this was a real kiss.

"What is rule one, Beck?" She needed to think of something other than how his mouth would feel against hers.

He raised an eyebrow.

"You said it before Minnow…" Violet bit her lip, then took a swig of her drink. Veterinarian work was incredibly rewarding. Unfortunately, it could also be devastating— particularly for those who worked in emergency med. The hard cases stayed with you.

"Right." Beck shook his head. "Rule one is I never plan to marry. Or at least not until I am old…like thirty-five." It was his standard statement and joke. The thirty-five was a number he and a friend had chosen in college. Nothing serious, but he saw the hurt flash across Vi's eyes.

"Damn it. Sorry, Vi. It's a joke. I always add the age, and I wasn't thinking and I…" Wow he was digging a hole but couldn't seem to get his brain to stop spitting words. "I don't think you are old."

"It's fine, Beck." Vi shrugged. "I thought thirty-five was old too when I was twenty-six. It seemed very far off. Then I blinked and." She gestured to herself.

The woman was fine. And not fine like everything is fine. But F-I-N-E. She was gorgeous and he'd just jammed his foot in his mouth.

"The good news is that I don't have any immediate plans to race to the aisle." She let out a sigh. "One failed trip to that altar is enough to make one supercautious. This is a fling, remember." She pulled his free hand into hers. Her fingers twisting through his.

Heat shot through him as her thumb traced circles on this wrist.

"So key chains?" He pulled her hand to his lips.

"Oh." Violet let out a giggle. "I have no idea how that happened but I love them. I used to pick one up every place I traveled. Now any that make me laugh come home with me. My collection is well over a hundred at this point."

"Nice. I don't really have a collection of anything. Well, coffee mugs. But those are holdovers from Mom, mostly." His father had bought any mug his mother wanted, and she'd wanted a lot of them. Silly phrases—yep. Innuendos—of course. Looked like it belonged in the trash already—she'd love it.

"I need another drink. A water this time. You want anything?" She squeezed his hand, then pulled back.

"I'll get it." Beck needed a moment to gather his thoughts. Find a way to make sure he didn't utter any more stupid jokes tonight.

Violet clapped as the singer finished the angry breakup song. The singer's girlfriends were all cheering in the booth next to them.

"No need to be a body language expert to know she is going through it." Beck squeezed her arm.

He'd slid into the side of the booth with her about an hour an ago. They'd chatted about their backstories and silly things. It was relaxing, despite his initial faux pas about age.

She let out a yawn and he smiled. "I think that might be our signal to call it a night."

"We can't. You lost the bet but if we leave now, it's a draw." She yawned again.

"We'll just have to table the bet for another night. You are exhausted, Vi."

Competition flared through her. She hadn't felt the bite of it for years. Since Thomas and she went their own ways. But the glow was there now.

"Come on." She grabbed his hand and pulled them out of the booth. She was winning the bet.

Heading toward the stage she quickly flipped through the book, found the number for "Monster Mash," and pushed the code into the machine. There were two mics, so she handed one to him and grabbed the other.

Beck was laughing. "Vi, I can't sing. I'm terrible at it."

"Well, then it is a good thing for you that this is karaoke night. No one is expecting perfection!"

The musical bars started playing, and she waited for the words to start appearing on screen. "I thought you always jumped at experiences."

Beck playfully threw a hand over his chest. "You wound me, dear lady."

Her laughter nearly made her miss the song's first words.

The three minute song was over too fast. As the music cut out the giggles started. "I guess I win."

"I guess you do." Beck took her mic, his fingers grazing her wrist.

She'd had exactly two beers in the three hours they'd been there. She was sober, but as his blue gaze met hers, she nearly swooned.

Two women stepped up to the book of available songs, and she grabbed his hand. "Come on, we have to go before their song starts or we both lose."

"I didn't realize you were so competitive." Beck wrapped an arm around her waist as they headed to the coat rack.

"I used to be really competitive. It was why I was such a good agility trainer. It made me feel alive." She slipped into her coat and waited for Beck to grab his.

The bars of the next song were starting as they hit the door, but the words hadn't started, so she was going to keep the win.

She walked to her car. The night was cool, but compared to what was coming in the next few weeks, it was balmy. Something her Florida friends would not have agreed with.

"So since I won the bet, do I get to kiss you or you kiss me? We never actually spelled out the terms, which looking back at it was an oversight." She was giddy. Violet couldn't remember the last time she felt like this.

No, she could. Her bachelorette party. They'd danced on tables, at a location where that was allowed. It was an experience and she'd jumped at it. Easily.

She hadn't been that person in so long.

"I think as the winner you get to decide. Do you want to kiss me?" He leaned against the door of her SUV, his gaze never leaving hers. "Or do you want me to kiss you?"

Her brain short-circuited. Both options were amazing. Both options heated her skin. There was literally no wrong answer.

Violet looked toward the entrance of the bar as a couple walked out laughing. She missed that kind of companionship. The excitement of someone next to you.

This was a fling. Something fun. But even the idea of it was awakening something she'd kept dormant since forever.

"I want you to kiss me." Violet held up her head, expecting Beck's lips to capture hers immediately.

Instead, he leaned his arm against her SUV. Then he put his other arm around her waist. His sweet, honeyed gaze swept over her. Sounds echoed around them as others headed to their cars, but they were far away. Like somehow, Beck had slipped them into a world all their own.

His fingers spread on her back as he looked at her. "You are so perfect." The arm on the SUV drew the loose hair away from her eyes.

"Beck." She breathed out his name. Violet had never had someone stare at her as though nothing else in the world mattered. As though they could look at her forever and never tire of the image.

Her knees felt like they might buckle and heat filled her cheeks. "Kiss me."

This time, he didn't hesitate. His lips brushed hers, then the hand on her back pulled her closer and he deepened the kiss.

There was nothing rooting her to the ground. Everything in this moment was Beck. Her mouth opened and his tongue grazed hers. His hands ran up and down her back, drawing her even closer.

Her body crashed to the ground as he pulled back.

"I had fun tonight, Vi." He wasn't kissing her, but his arms still held her tightly.

"Me, too. We'll have to come back here sometime." The words spilled out and she bit her lip. This was a fling. Kisses and a date to a wedding. It wasn't a plan anything kind of relationship.

"I'd like that." Beck kissed the top of her head, then stepped back. "Have a lovely evening, Vi."

CHAPTER FOUR

BECK STRETCHED BEFORE he walked into the clinic. He was going to see Vi. At work.

That last part was important. This was work. The place they were keeping separate. It was something they'd agreed on the other night at Don's. At work they were colleagues.

When the fling was over, they still had to work together. He'd readily agreed, but that was before he'd kissed her. The taste of her had lingered for hours. Or maybe his brain had just latched on to the perfection that was Vi and refused to let the happiness go.

As he walked into the clinic he waved to Lacey, then headed toward the back room. The receptionist was wearing cat ears. Halloween was still more than three weeks away, but Lacey loved the holiday and started dressing up as different animals on October 1. The cat ears were actually pretty tame compared to her usual monthly attire.

"Hi, Beck." Violet was looking in on Patches, a small dog that had come in the same night as Minnow. Patches was dehydrated for reasons they hadn't been able to figure out.

Looking over Vi's shoulder, he couldn't stop the smile. Patches was wagging her tail and standing right by the door of her enclosure.

"Someone looks better."

"Right." Vi turned. Her dark hair was up in a messy bun

today, and she was grinning from ear to ear. "Her panels came back clean, so I think it was a viral infection."

"You gave your parents a very big scare, little one." Beck wagged a finger at the enclosure. Patches offered a yip and more tail wags.

"Right." Vi shook her head. "I told her the same thing. The good news is they are on their way to get her. Happy times."

"Those are the best times." Beck leaned against the counter. "Did you see Lacey's cat ears? Is it wrong that the easiness of today's costumes makes me wonder what we will see her in on Halloween?"

Vi shook her head. "No. I asked her what her costume is for Halloween and she said it was a secret. I reminded her that Halloween tends to be very busy and she needs to be able to move easily."

"So no giraffe repeat?" Last year Lacey had barely been able to get into the office with the papier-mâché head she'd built for the costume.

"Right." Violet moved over to the other pup they'd been monitoring for several days. Patches looked significantly better; Nix did not.

The gray cat was curled up in a ball in the back of the enclosure. He barely lifted his head when Violet reached in.

"His panels are also back. Kidney disease."

Given the cat's advanced age, that didn't surprise Beck. It still sucked.

"I already let Linda know. She bought some beds so he is more comfy since jumping up into her bed is harder now. She is going to switch his food and just love on him for as long as possible." Vi rubbed Nix's head. The cat let out a low purr but didn't raise his head.

The pager on his hip buzzed. "Looks like the first patient

of the night is here." Beck sent a silent hope up that such an early arrival didn't mean they were in for a long night.

He stepped into the room to see a young woman holding a small dog. The little guy was shaking, and Beck blinked twice. The black dog had a stripe on his nose and a white patch on his chest. The dog looked just like his childhood pet, Lolly.

He took a deep breath and offered a smile to the worried pet parent. "I'm Beck, the vet tech. What brings you in tonight?"

"My mom brought over my gran's rocking chair." She let out a soft sob. "Gran passed last month and I love the rocker."

"Of course." Beck nodded. The dog looked like it was in pain, but it wasn't bleeding. If the woman didn't get to the point shortly, he'd redirect her.

"I was rocking in it. Remembering Gran. I had my eyes closed and—" she let out a sob "—the next thing I heard was Bug screech."

She bit her lip so hard, Beck feared she was tasting blood.

"Okay. Do you know what part of Bug was under the rocking chair?"

"His tail."

Beck took a step closer and Bug snarled at him. Not an unexpected reaction. Small dogs were notoriously feisty despite their size, and an injured animal was always more prone to strike first and ask questions later.

"I am going to muzzle Bug so I can get a good look at him." Beck pulled the muzzle out of the cabinet.

The owner held up her hand and he prepped himself to explain why muzzles were good for Bug and the staff. "I can do it. I've muzzled him at our regular vet before. He isn't a full Chihuahua, but he has many of their traits."

She took the muzzle from his hand, got it on Bug, then

gently passed her little boy over to him. It was easy to see the damage to the tail.

"Oh. You poor guy." Beck spoke softly to Bug, even as the tiny dog voiced his obvious displeasure at being held, the muzzle and his tail. "I am going to take Bug to get X-rays. Dr. Lockwood will want to see what is happening there."

The woman let out a soft sob and curled into herself.

As he started toward the door, Beck turned. "This isn't your fault. Promise."

"Lacey says Nola is having a cup of tea, but she doesn't want to leave until after the surgery is completed." Violet looked at Bug's X-rays one more time. The rocking chair had crushed his tail almost at the base.

Tail crushes weren't always an emergency. Sometimes they could give the pup pain meds and do surgery during regular business hours. But X-rays indicated Bug's tail crush was causing nerve damage. The longer the pressure was on the nerve, the more likely Bug was going to suffer long-term consequences.

She turned and looked at Beck. He was bent over Bug, carefully monitoring the dog's breathing. "How is Bug?"

Beck looked up and nodded. "Good. He is fully under, and his heart rate is staying steady."

"Excellent." Violet went to the sink, washed up and donned gloves. "I hate having to amputate his tail, but that nerve damage might hurt his back."

"He will be the cutest boy with the bobtail. Then he really will look just like my Lolly." Beck rubbed a gloved finger over Bug's ear.

"Lolly?" Violet stepped to the table and picked up the scalpel. She took one quick breath before starting the surgery.

"Lolly was my puppy growing up. I found her at the university behind a garbage can when I was waiting for my dad to get out of a meeting. I was seven. Lolly was probably two or three. She had a bobtail and looked just like this guy." Beck tilted his head, and she knew he was seeing a dog he loved and had to say goodbye to.

"You had a small dog and now you have an agility border collie? Did you want a big dog and your parents wouldn't let you have one?" Her mother had been against having a dog.

"No. Lolly found me, and Toaster was too much for her first owner. Border collies don't do well in shelters. Destruction is their go-to the moment they are bored." It was nice that Beck was willing to have dogs of all sizes. She was partial to large dogs, but that didn't mean if the right small pup showed up, she wouldn't jump at that opportunity too.

Nope. That mental thought felt a little too close to seeing a future. They were having a fun fling. Rushing into thoughts like that was how she'd gotten stood up at the aisle years ago. She shouldn't need the reminder.

"Did you parents do agility?"

It shouldn't be an awkward question, but then so much about growing up she found awkward as an adult. The stories she'd told as family lore—fights over coats, or learning to climb onto the top of the fridge when her parents were arguing so if any glass got broken she didn't step on it, or that time her mom asked her dad to pick her up and she got left at school because he swore she hadn't asked and neither wanted to admit the other was right—weren't as silly as she'd thought they were.

"No. My mom didn't want a dog. I wanted one so bad. I asked for a puppy every year at Christmas from the time I was thirteen when Yoshi showed up under the tree. Mom was not pleased. She said the first time he did something bad it was right off to the shelter with him."

The memory of her starting to cry and her father starting to yell at her mother echoed through her soul. Her father had gotten the dog for all the wrong reasons. Her mother was heartless about anyone else's feelings. And she'd been a kid who'd just gotten warned she could lose her puppy anytime. Even with all that, it had still been her happiest Christmas.

"I trained him so there was no reason Mom could give to get rid of him. Then I found that I liked it."

Violet smiled behind her mask. "Yoshi and I won regionals, then youth nationals. I lost him when I was a senior in college. By then he'd stopped doing agility work and I was competing with Pebbles, but in a world of good boys, he was the bestest."

"You got into agility to keep your mom from giving away your dog?" It didn't matter that he was wearing a mask, she could see the frown through his eyes.

"My mom needed control. She got meds for anxiety after a breakdown about four years ago. It's better. Now, she lives in Arizona, owns her own pottery shop and is dating someone who I think makes her genuinely happy."

Now that her mother's mental health had been addressed, it hurt that the woman she was now would have been a good mother. That woman would have loved her dearly. Violet had forgiven her, but they would never be close.

"My father isn't exactly a saint in this story. He knew my mother didn't want an animal in the house. In her defense, he never helped with a lick of housework. The man was weaponized incompetence personified." Getting a puppy out of spite was pretty much the worst reason to get another living creature. The fact that it had worked out was due more to Violet's stubbornness than anything else.

"Wow."

She couldn't fault Beck for not having anything else to add to that conversation. "How often did your parents fight?"

Violet looked at the bone around the tail. Hoping to find a way to save more of it.

"Very rarely. I remember they argued once when Dad wanted me to join soccer. Or rather Dad was tired of me pestering him about me joining soccer. Mom didn't agree."

"The team too expensive?" Violet had played lacrosse and her parents had supported her, though they stood on opposite sides of the field when they attended games together.

"Too dangerous." Beck let out a chuckle that had little humor behind it. "All sports were too dangerous. I guess after finally having me, they weren't willing to risk losing me. But I never had to hop up on the counter to avoid flying glass."

"Oh." Violet frowned as the tail's full damage came into view.

"What's going on?" Beck looked at the array of displays showing Bug's status. "He is still holding on well. Heart rate steady. Breathing normal."

"The tail is shattered thoroughly at the base. I was hoping with the X-rays we might be able to give the guy a little more tail, but…" Disappointment spread through her as she got the instruments ready for the amputation.

"Bug won't even notice after it's healed. Dogs are incredibly resilient. Heck, I've heard more than one vet say they are three-legged animals with four legs. Losing his tail is unfortunate but hardly the end of the end of Bug's fun adventures."

She knew that. Beck was saying all the right things. A

dog's tail was technically an extension of its spine, but losing it wouldn't do any long-term damage.

"I just thought I might have some good news to deliver. Rather than we had to go farther up so the bobtail I talked to you about is more of a nub." She finished the amputation quickly.

So often in emergency vet medicine it was a tale of we tried this but had to do that. She always hoped for an unexpected "it was smoother than anticipated." Those were so few and far between.

"My dad once worked on an archaeology dig outside the Great Pyramid of Giza."

Violet didn't look up from closing the wound at the base of Bug's now tiny tail. But he had piqued her curiosity. "What? That is so cool."

"Yeah." Beck checked the oxygen mask they had over Bug's snout. "He had pictures that he kept in his office. He always said the pictures made it seem better. That he spent the summer shifting sand and finding nothing."

"Nothing?"

"Nothing. Dad wasn't in a very active dig. To quote him, he was helping to make sure nothing had been missed. And they confirmed that."

"Still. The experience." The old Violet had loved traveling. She'd made a habit of staying over after a competition ended to see the sights. Thomas had never understood, and eventually, she'd stopped.

Another little piece of herself she'd given up to a man who'd never really cared about her.

"You must have traveled to some amazing places with them." She finished up the final stitches, then used a sterile wash to clean the closed wound.

"Nope. They found each other. Settled down in Maine and never looked back. Dad used to say Mom was his greatest adventure."

Beck said the words as if on repetition. Just like she had stories she told over and over. He had the same.

"That is really sweet." To be loved so completely. That was all she'd ever wanted.

"Yes. And boring. They had these great lives, then they met each other, settled down and that was it. They could have had so much more." Beck shrugged. "You ready for me to start waking him?"

"Yes." She stepped back from the table, pulling off her gloves. "Is that why you don't want to marry until you are old? Like thirty-five or so?" She winked hoping to show him she didn't mind the faux pas from the other night.

"Thirty-five isn't old." He didn't look up from Bug as the dog started to come out of the sedation. The dog would be groggy all day, but animals awoke from sedation much quicker than humans.

"That wasn't an answer to the question." Except it was. She'd heard it the other night in his rule. Violet went over to the sink, washed up and turned to watch Beck finish bringing Bug out of his slumber.

"I just don't want to miss out on anything." He looked over his shoulder. "Like running away to Miami for a weekend with a hottie who wants to make her ex jealous."

She rolled her eyes, then headed for the door. She needed to let Bug's owner know that her boy was doing well, and the tail was going to be very short, but he would 100 percent recover. And she wanted a minute alone too.

Violet wasn't looking to race down the aisle. She was content enough in her town house with Bear. So why was there a tinge of regret brewing in her chest? This was a fling for fun and to save face at the wedding. It wasn't a life jump start.

CHAPTER FIVE

"LET'S GO, TOASTER!" Beck pushed sweat from his eyes as he ran his dog through the course again.

"Now that is the kind of dedication I want to see at this gym." Nancy beamed as she and Oliver stepped onto the agility course.

Beck raised a hand and motioned for Toaster to heel. His girl followed the command, her tail still wagging as they started off on the course. They were competing at regionals as part of the intermediate team. He'd love to say that he was here to make sure Toaster was ready to win, but he didn't care about the prize.

He was running off the emotions he'd created last night when taking care of Bug. Trying to push everything he'd felt for Vi into a cage in the back of his head. Preferably before she got here.

She'd promised him some pointers for Toaster before regionals. An off-handed comment she'd made after Bug's surgery that he'd taken quick advantage of. Again, not for the pointers, but to spend time with Vi.

Something about the way she'd asked if his parents' happy union and settling down was his reason for his *rule one*, made him uncomfortable. Violet hadn't pushed. Hadn't told him it was dumb to avoid marriage after witnessing such a happy union.

That was his college girlfriend's complaint. She'd been furious when they'd gone on a short trip for their one-year anniversary and to celebrate junior year finals and not come back engaged. She'd dumped him about three weeks later. Last he heard she was living in Colorado with her husband and a newborn. He wished her well, but she was the reason he set up rule one.

It was better to be up front about the expectation. That way no one got hurt. His life was full of adventures—the adventures his parents had given up in exchange for vows.

Vi accepted it. She didn't tell him he was a fool for not wanting what they had. So why was this the first time he felt odd about it? It was probably just…well, he didn't know why he was feeling like the rule might be wrong.

The feeling would pass.

"I need to run Oliver through the course. He's slow this week." Nancy pushed past him, Oliver trotting beside her.

He didn't bother to say anything to that. Nancy thought everything was slow except personal records, or PRs. The fact that PRs were rare, that Oliver was older now, that the course was something he knew so well he might be bored, were not considerations Nancy gave.

In her defense, the woman loved her dog; she just pushed toward prizes that never seemed to come.

"Beck." Violet waved as she stepped through the front door.

Nancy's head snapped. This private training session was about to get an uninvited guest.

"Dr. Lockwood." Nancy ran over, Oliver close at her heels.

"Hi." Vi nodded to Nancy as she stepped beside Beck.

He slid a hand around Violet's waist and kissed the top of her head. The simple motions sent flames down his spine.

Damn.

He had a serious crush on Violet. Getting to touch her, kiss her was igniting his feelings instead of dousing the flames.

"If you are going to be here, you must be a member. I know you came for the potluck as a date, but if you are going to be here for actual gym time…" Nancy put her hands on her hips.

"Members are allowed to sponsor people for a month, Nancy." He'd looked into it following the potluck. Vi had walked away from agility training. She was done with this life, and he had no plans to drag her back in.

"That sponsorship is for people bringing their dogs, Beck. Not trainers." Nancy crossed her arms—she really had the ticked-off owner bit down. "I must be firm, or others might try the same thing."

Lucky for her Vi had no desire to run her own agility gym. Nancy would be out of business tomorrow.

"Of course." Violet smiled.

The look he'd seen on her face at karaoke night was back. The competitor. The winner. Nancy had no idea who she was dealing with.

"Your website, which is outdated, indicates trainers are required to pay the monthly fee plus a sixty percent commission on all lessons." Violet reached into her back pocket, pulling out her phone. "Industry standard is forty percent to the gym."

"Well, I have all the clients here. So they are already gym members." Nancy raised her chin. "I am sure your fees will cover any expenses just fine. You *are* Violet Lockwood."

"I am." She hit a few buttons and held her phone up. An email was clear on the screen. "As you can see, I signed up as a trainer before coming in here. For the full year."

Nancy gave a little hop, then caught herself. "Lovely. We are happy to have you. I am sure whatever training schedule you set up will be very fruitful…for you."

It didn't take long for Nancy to see the dollar signs.

"I actually already reached out to the intermediate team. They will be here—" Violet turned her phone around and looked at the clock "—well, any minute, really."

"You are hosting a full training session." Nancy bit her lip, and if he and Vi weren't there, Beck figured she'd dance all the way back to her office.

"Yes. I already worked out the rate with them." Violet grinned, but he knew it was the smile she gave to pet parents she was furious with.

Tim, Lisa and Grace walked in, their dogs, Pickle, Tuna and Posy on leashes by their side. The handlers' grins dropped a little as they looked between Nancy and Violet.

"Hi, guys." Violet was a late-shift ER vet now, but when she'd arrived in Bangor, she'd been a regular shift vet and seen most of the dogs in the gym at some point. "Glad you could make it."

"Wouldn't miss this." Tim rubbed Pickle's ears. The border collie mix had gotten her name after eating nearly half a jar of pickles his daughter had drained and left out, for reasons the then-nine-year-old had not been able to explain.

Pickle had been seen in the office for an upset belly, but the puppy had been fine after a day or so. Tim had gotten her into training as soon as she was doing her business outside.

"Are you sure about the price?" Grace held on to Posy's leash. The pittie mix loved agility and was incredibly well trained. People were forever coming up to her, assuming her dog was a friendly beast.

"I am positive. Go ahead and give it to Nancy." Vi turned to the owner. "I am going to head out to the A-frame. Meet me there when you are done."

Nancy didn't bother to hide her glee. "We finally have Violet Lockwood as a trainer."

"I don't think she plans to do this very often." Lisa pulled a dollar out of her pocket and handed it to Nancy.

"What is this?"

"Our fee. Violet is doing it for a dollar." Lisa snapped her fingers and Tuna followed her onto the agility path.

"A-a d-dollar!" Nancy stuttered as each of the intermediate team laid a dollar in her hand then headed onto the field.

Technically, he hadn't worked out a fee with Vi, but he pulled out a dollar and passed it over too.

Round one to Violet.

"One more lap, everyone. Then we will call it a night." Violet wrapped her arms around herself as she watched the intermediate team run along the outside of the course with their owners.

The dogs had done the course at least twice but while speed was important, many wins came down to tuning everything but their owner out during the competition. Competitions were noisy. Busy. Filled with a million different scents. It was a dog's dream and a trainer's nightmare.

"Come on, Oliver." Nancy was racing Oliver through the course for at least the fifth time.

Violet had not appreciated Nancy's tone when she came with Beck for the potluck. She'd looked at the contract for trainers and started steaming. Beck had said Nancy complained about the lack of agility trainers at the gym. But she was doing nothing to court them.

There was a gym in New Port about thirty minutes away. It had two trainers; one she knew lived in Bangor. But that gym practiced industry standards of 40 percent for established members of the gym. If the trainer brought the client in, the trainer kept 80 percent.

Why would they work at Nancy's gym? Violet didn't plan to really do a lot of training, but it was the principle.

She blinked. She didn't *plan* to do any training. Tonight was a one-off. She'd explained that to Tim, Lisa and Grace. A quick hit to get Toaster fully integrated into the team. Regionals was less than a month away.

The team might not care if they came away with trophies, but they needed to be a team. It was safest for the dogs and their handlers if they acted as one. Though even with this brief interaction it was clear Toaster was going to run with them just fine.

Heck, with a little bit of work they might even place. Not win…though with a lot of work that was not outside the cards. The dogs were all super fit; and most importantly they all loved to run the course. That was one of the biggest indicators of success.

A factor many in the game overlooked. A fast dog only won if it was motivated. You could motivate through routine—not her favorite. Through fear—an absolute nonstarter for her. But nothing motivated an animal like fun.

"You are amazing." Beck wrapped an arm around her shoulders. "Worth so much more than a dollar."

She kissed his cheek. "I appreciate you saying so. I used to charge a hundred dollars an hour."

"Only a hundred?" Beck raised that eyebrow.

"You sound like my ex. He got so upset that I only charged a hundred, unless—" She bit her lip and cleared her throat.

"Unless?" Beck squeezed her shoulder as they started toward the locker area.

"Unless it was clear they were only there for me personally." She let out an involuntary shake. "Thomas used to plaster my face all over our social media sites. He bragged that my beauty drove so much business."

It was creepy. But more, it was infuriating; it diminished her talent. Most of her clients came to her because they wanted *her* to train their dogs so that they won. Not because she was a pretty face.

Thomas had huffed more than once about her unwillingness to wear a full face of makeup with her hair done while she was training. He had not understood her reasons about comfort and heat—or more likely he just hadn't liked them. With time—and some therapy—she'd finally concluded he liked the idea of her more than her.

"I take it some of the men who showed up weren't interested in agility." Beck didn't even bother to make that sound like a question.

"A few showed up without a dog. I actually took one guy's money. I told him it was three hundred an hour that time, and then ran him through the course for an hour and a half. He was not pleased."

"Why didn't he just leave?"

Violet let out a laugh that she knew had no humor. "Because then he would have had to admit that he was there to try to sleep with me."

Beck leaned against the lockers, letting his hand graze Toaster's head. "And your at-the-time-fiancé didn't bother to step in? He was a trainer. He could have run the session or sent the guy packing."

He could have. But Thomas was more excited that because he'd stayed for the extra thirty minutes, that meant they got to charge him six hundred dollars. That was the night she should have walked away from her engagement. Should have packed her things or better yet, packed his and kicked him to the curb.

But she'd believed in fairy tales then. Had wanted the fairy tale so bad. Still did. But that want was never going to blind her again.

"It wasn't his style." She knew the words were clipped; knew Beck knew too.

His head bounced back just a hair, but the smile never faded. His dimples were certainly easy to look at.

"Why don't we stop for coffee? We can get Toaster a pup cup. She has certainly earned it." Beck pushed off the locker and offered her a hand. "My treat since you refused to take an actual paycheck for training the team tonight. But you have to admit one thing."

His dimples deepened. If she was ever going to swoon it was over dimples like his.

"What?"

"You had fun tonight."

"Of course." Vi wrapped her arm through his elbow. "You are very fun to be around, Beck."

"I am." He dropped a kiss on her forehead.

"And so modest." She playfully hit his hip with hers. "Modesty is certainly one of your top characteristics."

"So glad you see that. But I wasn't talking about fun with me."

Her steps didn't falter but her heart dropped. That last line stung. She'd had fun *with* him.

"You enjoyed being back on the course. Enjoyed the agility work. I know Bear has no desire to run a course but you—you like being here."

No. She loved being at the agility gym. Violet drank in the energy the owners got from racing through obstacles.

She came alive when a pup jumped in its owner's arms at the end, tail wagging. Knowing it was the bestest girl or boy in that moment.

But this was part of her past.

It doesn't have to be.

Her chest tightened as they headed to the exit. She'd joined. Yes, to prove a point to Nancy. But she was a member…and a trainer…for a year. She could come back anytime.

Violet had to do her best not to turn and look back before the door closed.

CHAPTER SIX

THE CLOCK WAS ticking down. Twenty-four hours before they landed in Miami. Did they know enough? Was the rouse going to work? They still had enough time to call it off. Enough time for her to own up to Fiona that she and Beck weren't a real couple.

Sure they'd been on a coffee date and to a karaoke bar. But could you really call training, coffee, and bad singing with a kiss in the parking lot dating?

No.

And the kiss. He hadn't kissed her after their coffee date. Hadn't asked if he could. Hadn't brought it up at all.

That shouldn't bother her. It didn't bother her.

Sure, Vi. You keep telling yourself that.

Her phone pinged.

The pic Fiona sent of herself next to a dress bag holding her wedding gown with a thumbs-up and a glass of champagne sped up the ticking of the clock in her head. Twenty-four hours!

Before Violet could respond, another text popped in.

Can't wait to meet your boyfriend. You haven't even sent me a picture. The text ended with a frowny face emoji.

Violet looked up to where Beck was looking over some results on the computer. She bit her lip, then snapped a quick photo.

Pulling it into the chat, she hesitated. "Beck."

He looked up, pushing his glasses up his nose a little. Damn. That was the photo she should have gotten. Hot vet tech with glasses. Real, nerdy, hottie aura going on.

Heat raced across her skin. Man, she'd never thought she had a type, but…

"Did you need something, Vi?"

"Yes. Sorry." She'd gotten lost in her own thoughts. Of him. "Fiona is texting."

"Getting cold feet?"

The question hovered between them.

"Nope. She loves Patrick. They could have gotten hitched at a busted-up courthouse, with no one they knew watching, and she'd have been on cloud nine to be his wife." That was another red flag she'd missed.

Thomas had wanted a fancy wedding. He'd insisted on having a top caterer. The best photographer they could afford. The demands were ironic considering he'd seen none of it, but they'd had to pay for everything.

"That is the way it should be. My parents were married at the courthouse as soon as they got back to the States. My dad used to joke that his parents found out about my mom the day after they'd made everything legal." Beck's eyes closed for a moment as he clearly relived a happy time.

It was weird how he was so insistent on putting marriage off when he'd come from a happy home. She'd come from the exact opposite and had wanted the union so badly.

"She wants a photo of you. I snapped one while you were looking at Pi's results. I was going to just send it but that felt like such an invasion of privacy and…" Her words seemed to run off.

"Let me see it." Beck stepped up and looked at the photo.

He was bending over and you could see the pensive look on his face, his glasses just a little down his nose.

"You captured my best side."

"What?"

"My backside. I've heard my butt is quite delicious." Beck crossed his arms, giving her a look full of glee.

If she said it wasn't his best side it would be a lie. If she said it was, she admitted to focusing on his butt.

"I thought you said your right side was your best side? You were very insistent as I recall." She pursed her lips to keep the laughter in.

Beck's dimples popped out, and she mentally snapped that picture. "Touché."

"But that isn't the photo you should send." He pulled his phone out of his pocket.

It took a second, but her phone dinged and she looked at the adorable photo of him and Toaster at the agility park. It was perfection.

She quickly forwarded it to Fiona, then bit her lip. "Care to take a selfie of us to send, too?"

"You bet!" He wrapped an arm around her shoulders, his dimples showing so perfectly in the photo.

Violet snapped the photo and sent the picture off. "So, do Pi's results show a skin infection?" She already knew the answer. Or rather she was 90 percent certain she knew.

"No." Beck blew out a breath. The fun demeanor shifting away in an instant. "No mites. No bacteria. No fungus. Perfect skin."

Which meant the herding dog was pulling out his fur because of OCD. It was something she'd seen before. It was more common in working dogs, but any dog could develop it.

"Did Margery mention how long it's been since Pi's been

in the field?" Margery ran a sheep farm, but the Australian cattle dog had been out of commission due to a foot injury for at least a month.

Every dog had a purpose. Her Bear's purpose was to laze around, give snuggles, eat as much as possible and fart at the most inopportune moments. A cattle dog's main purpose was to herd cattle.

She'd seen herding dogs who needed to retire because of age or injury who adjusted to live as a house pet easily...or semi-easily. Often, they took to herding other animals in the house or the children.

Other herders never adjusted to a new life.

"All right, let's go talk to Margery." Violet took a deep breath. In many ways the best answer would have been mites, or even a hard-to-treat fungal infection. Mental health issues were hard enough to treat in humans where you could have an actual conversation. In animals, it could be a life-long challenge.

Pi was pacing the room as they walked into the small suite where Margery was waiting. The older woman was holding her arms as she stared at Pi. Tears ran down her cheeks as she looked over at Violet and Beck.

"It's OCD, isn't it? Not a fungal infection or mites." She ran the back of her hand over her cheeks.

Some people had a misconception that people who had working dogs didn't care about them as much as people whose dogs' whole purpose was just to love them. It wasn't true.

"Yes." Violet set her tablet chart on the counter and stepped over to Margery as she let out a sob.

"Pi stepped on a rock three weeks ago. He saw Dr. Brown who diagnosed a sprained tendon. Pi needs rest, but he won't accept it. But he is still favoring that back left leg. If I let him herd the sheep, he might tear the tendon. If I don't, he paces nonstop in the house." Margery let out a sob as she watched Pi continue to circle the room.

"I've got food puzzles and interactive play toys but…" She shrugged. "He isn't interested in any of that."

That wasn't a surprise. Cattle dogs were bred to herd. It was an instinct. She often warned new pet parents that you could train a dog, and you should, but you couldn't train the innate breed characteristics out of them.

"I think our best option is to get Pi on a low dose of serotonin reuptake inhibitors."

"You mean SSRIs?" Margery bit her lip as she watched Pi continue his rounds. "I am on a low dose of Prozac for anxiety and seasonal affective disorder."

"Yes. I mean SSRIs. Sometimes, just like with humans, the brain needs a little help. Once Pi gets back into the field the symptoms will probably subside, but you should come back during regular business hours to see Dr. Brown if they don't."

"Probably won't." Margery gave her a watery smile. "I know I pay an upcharge for after-hours emergency care but getting here during regular hours hardly ever works out. And Pi likes you." She double clicked the training clicker she had in her hand. Pi came, sitting at her feet before looking up at her.

The dog was focused. Too focused.

"All right. I will get the prescription written up and our in-house pharmacy can fill it. I want to warn you that SSRIs take time to build up in the system. You won't see the full effect from them for a month. But I want you to follow up after six weeks."

"If Pi is not back in the field by then, both of us will be beside ourselves." Margery rubbed the dog's ears.

"Understandable." Beck turned to grab some of the patient education materials they kept in the cabinet.

As she headed through the door to the back of the clinic, she heard him carefully going over the medication and then offering some of his own tricks for dealing with a dog with high drive needs.

The man was born to work in this field.

"Why the frown?" Beck had taken too much pleasure in Vi sending a pic of them to her friend. This was a fun fling. They were enjoying dates, and they'd shared a few kisses. There was hardly a significant reason for his heart to have floated when he looked at the selfie of them she'd sent to Fiona.

"Oh." Violet looked up from her phone. "Fiona says we make a great couple."

He barely kept the frown off his face. This was what she wanted. What they were attempting to accomplish. Why was she upset that it was working?

And why am I upset that she isn't thrilled at the idea of her friend thinking we are great couple?

That was a worry for another day.

"She thinks we make a great couple from a photo. And I mean... I am so glad you agreed to this, but now that we are taking off tomorrow morning... I... I..."

Rose coated her cheeks as she failed to find any words.

"Now you worry we are going to fall flat on our faces?"

"Yes." She looked relieved that he'd said what she was struggling to vocalize. They'd worked together for two years, but he'd always been able to fill in the blanks with Vi. It was a weird superpower that he'd joked about with the other vet techs only once.

He could still see their faces as he talked about how easy

it was to read her. How he could finish her sentences because she was an open book. The other vet techs had each shaken their heads and informed him that he was out of his mind.

Bethany, a vet tech who'd left the practice about six months ago, had flat out asked if he was sleeping with her. Because none of them could read Vi's mind. In fact, she worried constantly that Dr. Lockwood was mad at her because the woman was so quiet.

He'd clammed up quickly after that. Never sharing how easy it was for him around Vi. At least now that weird superpower came in handy.

"We have been on three dates. Everyone knows that if you make it to date four then things have a chance to get serious." Vi put her phone in her scrub pocket and headed over to where they were running tests on a puppy that had come in with what the owner swore was parvo, a devastating and highly fatal disease for puppies.

The rapid test had come back negative, and Violet was certain it wasn't parvo. But the patient's owner had insisted on the additional test.

"Everyone knows that? I thought it was the third date people chat about." As soon as the words were out, his face heated.

"That's just because so many people say they wait until the third date to sleep with someone. But I mean that isn't really that big of a deal. It's the fourth date, the one that can no longer be called 'testing' for a relationship that matters." Vi said the words with such ease.

His mouth was hanging open. Beck knew that. Knew that his brain was misfiring.

"And we haven't had that fourth date. We are asking people to believe we've been together six months and we haven't had a fourth date. I mean, I think people are going to suspect."

He wanted to say, so what if they do. It was how he really felt. They were people she rarely saw. Fiona wouldn't care. But if Vi cared, then he wanted this to work for her.

"How about we do our fourth date tomorrow morning?"

"That's sweet." She looked up from the lab work she was running on the puppy. "But we are supposed to be at the airport so early—at least when you work the late shift you don't have to worry too much about oversleeping the alarm."

So true. He actually planned to stay awake until they got on the plane, then catch some shut-eye.

"There are coffee shops in the airport. Let's get there, have a fourth date."

"Great. We can get into the nitty-gritty of what we want out of relationships and the future."

Luckily her head was bent over the test results so she didn't see him take a step back as those words hit him. He was getting into dangerous water here. Sure they'd shared kisses and had laughs together, but he'd been very clear that he had no intention of marrying and Vi… Vi wanted marriage.

Maybe she didn't say it. But one did not get that close to the altar with a walking red flag unless you wanted the fairy tale. He couldn't give it to her. But maybe he could help her practice so she was ready when the opportunity presented itself.

"Yeah." The word felt so hollow but he forced it out. "Yeah, that is exactly what I mean. So, fourth date at the airport coffee shop."

"That actually sounds pretty romantic." Vi met his gaze. "Good news. No parvo. Bad news, we don't know why Tofu is so lethargic."

She crossed her arms as she leaned against the counter. "Pluses, no blood in the stool, no parasites and the lethargy isn't terrible—yet." Violet took a deep breath. "Negatives, vomiting, diarrhea and Tofu was the runt of the litter. Mom has had little interaction with the guy, and Billy's daughter is supplementing feeding."

"What is his daughter supplementing with?" Alarm bells were going off in Beck's head.

"Billy says he bought canned puppy formula so I assume that." Vi tilted her head. "What are you thinking?"

"When I was in school, we had a puppy present with similar digestive issues. The owner was giving the puppy cow's milk as a substitute for the mother not making enough for the litter of seven she had. It caused severe digestion issues."

"But if they have canned puppy supplement?" Vi shook her head. "I can't imagine why they would also use cow's milk."

"Billy's daughter is a teen. Sometimes they do things that don't make sense. This is a long shot, but there are no parasites and the parvo is negative. Our puppy got so sick, its kidneys shut down before the vet figured out what was going on. The little guy is a big guy now and doing fine last I heard, but it was touch and go for a while." Maybe he was barking up the wrong tree but this was plausible.

And they had nothing else to go on.

"Let's ask." Vi grabbed the test results she knew Billy would want to see and headed toward the door.

"It's not parvo."

Beck was always impressed that Violet didn't wait to deliver good or bad news. He enjoyed working with Dr. Brown, but the man tried to lay the groundwork for each diagnosis. It was his way of being helpful, but Beck had seen more than one pet parent start to panic as they waited for the actual results.

Billy rubbed Tofu's ears but a tear slipped down his cheek. "I'm glad but then what? Because Tofu is tiny but mighty. She hasn't let being the runt slow her down at all."

"Is there any chance someone in your house is giving her cow's milk?" It was a gentle way to ask the question, but there was authority behind it.

"Cow's milk?" Billy squeezed his eyes shut. "Like from the grocery store cow's milk?" He opened his eyes. "Sorry. Dumb question I know."

"No. I know this is a unique ask." Violet offered a small smile.

Billy reached into his pocket and pulled out a cell. He put it on a speaker as it started to ring. It took a moment, but finally his daughter answered.

"Daddy? Is Tofu all right? Does she have parvo?"

"Alex, take a deep breath. No, she doesn't have parvo, but Dr. Lockwood is worried she might have gotten some cow's milk."

"Oh." The line went quiet, and all the adults in the room looked at each other.

"How much milk have you given Tofu?" Violet's words were soft, as she leaned over the phone. Not giving Billy's daughter a chance to shift her story was a good option. It wasn't that kids lied, it was that they often tried to make excuses and the webs spun into more and more, before they finally admitted the truth.

"The puppy milk cans were in the basement, and I was running late for school." She let out a cry on the other end of the phone.

"Alex!"

Vi held up her hand as Billy raised his voice. There was time for him to discipline and explain what consequences could happen, but right now they needed answers. It was amazing to watch this woman work.

"How much, Alex? I need to know so we can treat Tofu best."

A whimper carried across the line. "I have used it in the morning before school the last four days. But at night I was using puppy milk. I was."

"It never dawned on you to bring a can up from the basement at night when you went down…" Billy sucked in a deep breath.

"Did I kill Tofu?"

"No."

"No."

"No."

All three adults answered at the same time and Tofu lifted her head, gave her tail a tiny wag.

"We'll talk about this when I get home, Alex. But Tofu is going to be okay." Billy told his daughter he loved her, then hung up.

"The good news is digestive distress is much easier to treat than parvo. I am going to prescribe something to calm her stomach and let her rest for the next several days. Schedule a regular checkup for Monday or Tuesday with Dr. Brown. And give her lots of love."

"Thanks, Dr. Lockwood."

Violet headed through the door to the back and he followed.

"Nice work." She smiled as she grabbed the chart and filled out the information for the prescription. "I would never have asked about cow's milk."

"Glad to have helped. My parents would have grounded me for a month if I pulled something like that. I suspect Alex will get something similar."

"She's lucky Billy isn't the type to give away her dog like my mom would have." She shrugged lightly in a way that broke his heart. Did she really understand how sad her childhood had been? Sometimes he wondered.

Violet opened her mouth, but before she could say anything else, the three dings echoed again.

Another emergency. Damn!

CHAPTER SEVEN

BECK YAWNED AS he stood behind Violet in the security line at the airport. The sun wouldn't cross the horizon for a couple more hours, and he hadn't managed to get any shut-eye last night. The emergency had been a house fire.

The pup, Hemingway, had burns on his tail and was dealing with smoke inhalation. His kitty friend, Ben, had been found an hour later, severe burns on her paws. Both cuties were going to be okay, but it had made for an extremely long shift.

That was not going to derail him though. Exhaustion was a choice, and he planned to look as upbeat and excited as possible for this "fourth date."

She slipped her shoes off, and he grinned at her socks.

Violet followed his gaze and stretched her toes. "I found a place that puts anything you want on a pair of socks."

"And Bear's face is almost the perfect choice."

Vi's mouth opened, clearly ready to argue about the *almost perfect* words, but he reached down and yanked his tennis shoes off.

"Oh my gosh." Vi pointed at Toaster's face.

"Toaster *is* the best thing you can put on socks."

Violet put her hands on her hips and shook her head. "On that we will have to agree to disagree but—" she pointed to their feet "—great minds think alike."

They certainly seemed to. Matching animal socks was very couple-like. Even if they hadn't meant too.

He pushed their carry-on luggage forward and stood back while she headed through security. Then he followed.

"I can't believe you have Toaster on your socks." Vi chuckled as she slid the bright pink slip-on shoes back on.

"Why not? You have Bear on yours." He'd gotten the socks as a Christmas present last year. Although could you really call it a present if you bought all the gifts yourself?

He'd been alone for the holidays for two years now. His father had passed when he was a freshman in college. His mother had followed two years ago, though the dementia had stolen her before that.

It was weird to be alone so young, but he still made the cookies his father loved and stuffed his stocking for his mother. It was a little way to stay connected to his family.

"True. But most men probably wouldn't wear them or, if they did, they'd wear them at home."

Beck didn't know about that. He had several male friends he was sure would put their pets on socks. Hell, Marcus had a special hoody so his cat could be carried. It was the only way he managed to get anything done since the animal was so clingy.

"That is their loss. If a man let what others thought of him stop him from doing something he wanted to do, then he had no one to blame but himself. I actually have Toaster on three pairs of socks. I got a deal if I ordered more than two pairs." He grabbed their bags and pointed toward the coffee shop.

Then stopped and frowned. The lineup appeared to be never-ending. It seemed everyone on the first flight of the day was stopping here before heading to their gates.

The few seats the coffee shop had were already claimed. Well, they could take their coffee to the gate.

"Ugh." Vi looked at the line. "I think this is the universe's way of telling me no caffeine, so maybe there is some hope that I'll sleep on the trip down even though I'm stuck in a middle seat."

"Middle seat?" Beck wanted to kick himself. He'd meant to make sure they had two seats together. Even the high of going on an adventure was not enough to kick his brain into gear when he was so exhausted.

Vi had been stoic through all their cases last night, but he knew it weighed on her. Sometimes working in the veterinarian world simply sucked. There were no other words for it.

"Yeah. The only thing left on the flight are two seats in first class. So middle seat, here I come." She yawned, then hung her head a bit. "Sorry, I'm not the best travel companion right now."

It was five fifty in the morning. They'd worked a tough shift and had an early morning flight, with a connection in DC before reaching Miami. Now she was apologizing for not being what—perky?

Reaching over, he wrapped an arm around her shoulders. "I think you are an excellent travel partner. Let's go to the gate and just relax. I think we earned it after that shift."

Leaning her head against his shoulder, Violet let out a soft sigh. "It was rough. But today is a new day."

When they got to the gate, he set his bags next to hers, then made a quick excuse and headed to talk to the gate agent. With any luck, he could see about those two first class tickets or at least get her moved into first class.

"Good morning." Beck smiled at the gate agent.

"How can I help you?" The young man took a deep breath and put a smile on his face, but Beck could see the hesitation.

Airport brought out the worst in some people. During his

travels he'd seen more than one inexcusable attack on the gate agents who were just trying to do their jobs. "I'm heading to Miami for a wedding. My girlfriend is a bridesmaid. We purchased tickets separately, and she is stuck in a middle seat."

"The flight is sold out, except for two first class seats. I'm sorry, sir."

"I know. But I was wondering if I could use my points to upgrade us to first class, or just her, if I don't have enough. She's an emergency veterinarian. Last night's shift was a hard one, and I just want her to rest before she has to dive into wedding stuff for her friend."

The man looked over to where Violet stood waiting, then back at Beck. "You would be fine with her being in first class but not you?"

Beck waited for a moment. Was there more to that question? "I'm sorry. It's early and I haven't had any caffeine so I don't really understand the question. Of course, it's fine if only she can sit up there."

The man let out a soft chuckle. "I had a guy yesterday who bumped himself from a middle seat and left his wife, three-month-old and six-year-old in coach."

"What!" That was horrific.

"Exactly." The man rolled his eyes. "The things you see. Can I have your names?"

Beck provided them, and the attendant tapped out a few quick things on his keyboard. Beck's phone dinged once, then again.

The attendant smiled. "You're both in first class on both flights."

"Both? I don't think I have enough points for both flights. Can you just make it her all the way down?"

The attendant shook his head. "Nope. I didn't use the

points. I can upgrade at the gate for all sorts of reasons, and it's nice to have someone just be kind for a change. Have a great trip, sir."

"Thank you." He turned and headed back to Vi.

She was already holding up her phone as he took the seat next to her. "What magic did you just pull? First class on both flights!"

"No magic. I just asked if I could use my points."

"No. No. You are already doing so much, Beck. I can't ask you to use your points too."

Wrapping his arm around her shoulders, he kissed her forehead. Why couldn't he stop the little touches? A fling was fun—and he'd had more than one in the past few years. Women who'd he'd hung out with for a few months, enjoying their time together. But he'd never found himself reaching for them without thinking. Dropping little kisses here and there.

At least it would look more natural at the wedding if they acted this way.

"You didn't ask. I acted. And it doesn't matter because the agent had a real louse of a guy yesterday and more than a few irate customers over the course of his career, so just being nice before six in the morning was enough." He looked at his watch, debating if there was enough time for a coffee run.

Violet laid her head against his shoulder, and all thoughts of seeking out coffee disappeared. No drink was worth giving this up.

"Guess our coffee date is off then." Vi yawned and snuggled against his shoulder.

"We can still have it. Just here." He leaned his head against hers. His eyes were heavy but he didn't dare close them. "So, Miami. You exchanged sun and heat for Bangor's less sunny much colder climate. Think you will head back south eventually?"

Every once in a while he searched on the real-estate apps for property and for a moment considered selling the house and trying someplace new. But the memories of his parents; the happiness he'd had there. He wasn't ready to give the link to his parents up.

At least not yet.

"No." Vi giggled. "Don't tell that to any of my friends at the wedding. They won't believe you. I think the idea that anyone would trade in the sand and sun for snow and gray-filled winters is beyond them."

She wasn't planning to leave Bangor. That made him oddly happy.

"I don't think our winters are really gray." Beck had heard more than one person comment about how Maine was gorgeous in three seasons but that didn't override the bleakness of the fourth.

"They aren't."

He smiled at Vi's simple words.

"They are frozen, but there is a beauty that comes with first snowfall. It's a season for hibernation and relaxing and staying warm with friends." She let out another yawn. "There is no way I can stay awake on the first flight. I think the first-class amenities will be an absolute waste on me."

Beck yawned, too. "We will be able to stretch out—at least as much as one can on an airplane. Not a waste."

"Not a great date, either." Violet turned, her dark eyes holding his.

"It's unique. That's the definition of great in my opinion."

She pressed a kiss against his cheek. "You are too perfect."

"Good. That will mean we'll make a great impression at the wedding."

* * *

"What do you think?" Beck stepped out of the hotel bathroom dressed in a light brown linen suit with a dark mocha shirt underneath.

Damn.

Violet had to swallow the rush of desire as she stared at his perfection. They'd slept on both flights down. She was still a little tired, but Beck looked like he was fully recharged… and ready to go. "That suit looks lovely on you."

If the suit looked that delicious on him, she couldn't wait to see the tux on Beck's muscular form.

"Well, I have to keep up with my date." He gestured to her. "You look gorgeous. Drop-dead gorgeous."

Beck tilted his head in such an approving look that she felt her toes curl in the taupe high heels she'd chosen for the floral minidress. It was the first time she'd worn the dress she'd found in a boutique downtown. It came to the top of her thighs, had long sleeves and a high neck, and was covered in dozens of different flowers. It was colorful and sexy as hell.

She loved it the second she saw it on the mannequin. Loved it more when she stood in front of the mirror in the dressing room. It had taken her over a year to have a reason to wear it, but it was worth it to see the look on Beck's face.

"Thank you." She'd sent a picture of herself to Fiona in the dress. It showed off Violet's long legs. It was a statement piece, but this wasn't her wedding. She wanted to make sure she approved. Fiona had sent back that if Violet didn't wear it to the rehearsal, she'd take it as a personal affront.

Beck held out his elbow. They were meeting the rest of the wedding party in the hotel lobby to take the party bus to the Frost Museum of Science. "Ready?"

"Yes." She smiled up at him. It was nice having him here. Yes, they were playing a game, but Beck was fun to be around.

He called her Vi and laughed with her. He paid attention and cared about people.

And he kissed like an absolute god.

She was getting ready to support Fiona as her bridesmaid and friend. But she was also about to see the man she'd foolishly expected to spend the rest of her life with. She should feel more nervous about that, but on Beck's arm it was impossible to feel self-conscious.

Her heels put her at the perfect height to place a kiss on his cheek. He'd held her in the airport. Kissed her forehead several times. It should feel weird to kiss him. Awkward to share the little touches partners did without thinking.

Instead it felt oddly…right.

Violet wasn't sure what to do with that, but that was a problem for future Violet. This weekend was going to be fun. Period.

They headed to the elevator bank, and all the good vibes they'd had seemed to get sucked out of the universe as she came face-to-face with a woman who looked remarkably like her.

"Wow." Beck blew out a breath.

He pulled her a little closer as the woman she knew must be Thomas's wife stared at her. The woman's hair was a shade lighter, her features a little softer than Violet's but the resemblance was uncanny.

She was wearing a knee-length yellow dress with a deep décolletage, paired with a teardrop amethyst necklace. One identical to the piece Thomas had given her for their first anniversary.

Cringe thy name is Thomas.

Awkward did not begin to describe the interaction as the two stared at each other.

"You have a doppelgänger." Beck chuckled but she could see him look above the elevator, probably hoping it would arrive so that whatever was going on ended quicker.

Unfortunately Violet knew the woman was getting on the party bus with them. The only saving grace was that Thomas wasn't with her.

"You must be Violet."

She smiled, grateful that Beck pulled her a little closer. He might not know exactly what was going on, but the man could read a room.

"I am. I apologize, but I don't know your name."

The woman lifted her hand, fingering the teardrop necklace. "Mrs. Dove Lowerly."

"It's nice to meet you." The waves of emotion she'd expected failed to crest. Maybe she would get through this weekend unscathed.

"Violet."

Nope. Her body tensed, and Beck squeezed her waist again as Thomas stepped around them and next to his bride.

"Hi, honey." He pressed his lips to Dove's. The motion was not gentle. It lacked love—in her opinion.

He'd done the same thing to her when he wanted people to understand she was with him. One of the red flags she'd ignored. Now he was doing the same to Dove.

Fury pulled at her, but Dove wrapped her arms around Thomas's neck, leaning into the possessive intent. If she was unbothered by the domineering attitude, then it wasn't Violet's place to interfere.

The elevator finally arrived. Thomas and Dove stepped in. Beck hugged her gently as they stepped in.

"So who are you?" Thomas started as soon as the door

closed. His eyes were trained on Beck. It was a look he'd give competitors on the agility course.

It wasn't appropriate there and it certainly wasn't appropriate here.

"Beck Forester." He kissed her head. "And you?"

Thomas let out a slow chuckle. "I think you know who I am."

Beck tilted his head, looked at her, then shrugged. "Sorry. No. Should I?"

Violet turned her head into Beck's shoulder, glad she had a matte, no-smear lipstick on because there was no way to keep herself from laughing if she had to look at Thomas. And Beck's suit was too perfect to ruin with bright red lipstick.

He was sputtering. And she knew from standing at his side for far too long that his cheeks were going from pale to fire-engine red. It was something he hated about himself but couldn't control.

"Thomas Lowerly." The words were curt. Spit out. "I am sure *that* clears it up."

"Sorry, it doesn't ring a bell. Are you old friends?"

The elevator door opened before Thomas could say anything else. She could not have scripted a better first meeting with Thomas.

"Come on. I have to introduce you to Fiona. She is going to love you." Violet kissed Beck's cheek, then pulled him out of the elevator.

This was a new experience, and she was going to enjoy every minute.

"So how did you and *Violet* meet?" Thomas crossed his arms as he stood next to Beck.

The groomsmen were lining up for the rehearsal. Beck had

hoped the man would avoid him and Violet after the uncomfortable elevator ride. Apparently not.

"Vi and I work together."

"You don't look old enough to be a vet."

"I'm not a vet. I'm a vet tech specialist." He ignored the smirk on Thomas's face. He'd gotten his degree, then a specialty license in emergency and critical care. He was very content with the career he'd chosen.

"But not a doctor of veterinarian medicine." It wasn't a question. It was clear from the glee on Thomas's face that he was happy Beck was "only" a vet tech.

His parents had doctoral degrees in their chosen fields, and they'd often reminded him that it just meant they'd spent more years in school and focused on something very specific. It didn't mean they were better than anyone else that they got to have "Dr." in front of their names.

"Are you a doctor?" Beck didn't actually care, but he took a little too much satisfaction in seeing the man's smirk fall away.

"No. Trainer. And business owner." He cleared his throat as the music started.

Violet was standing at the front of the procession, a bouquet of paper flowers in her hands. She was smiling and took a moment to find him. She offered a saucy little wink and Beck chuckled.

"She do any training in Bangor?" Thomas's question was low and barely audible.

Beck wanted to pretend not to hear it, but the man beside him was certainly capable of starting a scene. This was Fiona and her fiancé's night. A fact that should be easy for Thomas to understand as the stepbrother of the groom.

"Not really. She is focused on emergency medicine." The one practically free training lesson she'd given the intermediate team wasn't much. She'd had fun. So much fun, but her focus was her veterinary practice. That made sense; Vi had worked hard to become a vet.

He looked around wondering if there was a way to move to another seat. Not without turning a few heads. So he stayed where he was.

Luckily, the man seemed content to keep his mouth shut for the rest of the short ceremony. As soon as Violet walked down the aisle on the arm of a groomsman as the last bridesmaid to leave, Beck stepped around Thomas and followed his date.

He had no intention of fueling any discussion with the man. He was here for Vi. And she was getting what she wanted this weekend. So he'd deal with the nosy ex, but only when he had to.

"Isn't this venue amazing?" Violet's eyes lit up as she looked at the tank of jellyfish floating next to them.

"Yeah. I've never seen a wedding and reception in a museum before." When the party bus had pulled up to the Frost Museum of Science, Beck had looked around to see if there was some other venue he was missing, but no. The bride and groom were getting married under a thirty-plus-foot oculus with sharks and schools of colorful fish swimming by. Then the reception was going to be in The Deep, an aquarium area that was filled with tanks and portholes.

It was unique and fun but standing next to Vi was the best part of this adventure.

"Fiona has an aquatic medicine certificate, and Patrick is a marine biologist focused on conservation efforts. The two of them make the perfect team. Look." She held up the bouquet she'd used at the rehearsal.

It was paper flowers with marine life on them. "Wait, are those—"

"Yep. Fiona took the brochures people put in the recycle bin at the exit of the science museum and made all of our bouquets out of them. We are supposed to give them to her so she can compost them."

"Impressive." He'd never thought much about marriage. The few friends he'd seen tie the knot had all settled down into quiet married life. There were even babies starting to arrive now.

It was sweet, but at twenty-six, he wasn't ready to settle into a quiet matrimonial life. His parents had traveled the world, had experiences documented in large photo albums that he'd thumbed through so often they were cemented in his memory.

And every single one of those fun moments had ended right after they'd said their vows. He didn't doubt they'd been happy, but it was like they'd closed a chapter of their lives when they married. A chapter he was not ready to seal shut.

"Yeah. She is so much fun. Now it is dinner and dancing time. You up for it?"

She hit his hip with hers. It seemed to be something she did without thinking, a little touch for fun.

He liked it. A lot.

Pulling her close, he ran a thumb down her cheek, then pressed a featherlight kiss to her lips. They were supposed to be boyfriend and girlfriend after all. "I'm up for anything with you."

Color bloomed on Vi's cheeks, and she looked down as she shook her head. "Anything covers a lot."

"It sure does."

"You make her glow. I haven't seen that…ever." Fiona held out a drink to him as she looked out at the rest of the rehearsal dinner guests.

"I think it's the bride who is supposed to glow." Beck took the drink she offered and raised it toward her. "And you do. Congratulations."

"Thank you." Fiona grinned, but the look in her eye gave him a moment's pause. "But we aren't talking about me."

"It's the night before your wedding." One of Beck's friends had ended an engagement with a woman because she was so focused on the wedding, he'd feared she had no interest in the life that came after. A proven concern when she walked down the aisle not even a year later and filed divorce papers before the first anniversary.

Most brides weren't focused only on the wedding, but the night before they walked down the aisle it was, understandably, their primary concern.

"We have our marriage license and an officiant approved to sign said license in the State of Florida. After tomorrow I'll be Patrick's wife. Everything else is just icing on the cake."

Fiona took a sip of her drink never letting her eyes leave his. "But what I want to talk about right now, before Violet gets back from the bathroom, is you."

Beck let out an uncomfortable chuckle. "Is this where you tell me if I hurt her, you'll hunt me down?"

The bride tilted her head. "Do you need me to tell you that? Are you planning to hurt her?"

"Of course not!" Maybe the words were said too fast for someone who'd offered to pretend to be a long-term boyfriend but only offered a fling. That didn't change the facts. He had no intention of hurting Violet. Period.

They were having fun.

"Good." Fiona raised a brow as she took another drink.

She didn't say anything else, didn't ask how they'd met or

how long they'd been dating. If he had to make a guess, she understood exactly how long he'd been in the picture.

"Fiona." Violet was smiling as she joined them, but her focus was directed completely on the bride. "Are you keeping Beck company?"

"Yes. We were just getting to know each other." Fiona shrugged as she looked at him, a dare in her eye for him to offer any kind of disagreement.

She leaned over and kissed Violet's cheek. "I need to see to a few more of the guests. But no one is using the dance floor. I know how much you like dancing."

"You do?" Those were the wrong words.

Fiona let out a giggle and shook her head as she walked away. "She does."

"I don't think she buys our story. I'm sorry, Vi."

She looked over at the dance floor, then back at him. "I don't think Fiona was ever going to buy this. But I'm glad you're here, whether anyone believes this—" she gestured between them "—or not."

"Want to dance?" He set his drink on the high table next to him and held out her hand.

Violet beamed as she put her hand in his. "Hell yeah!"

They scooted out onto the dance floor, his hand holding hers up in the air. She was already swishing to the beat as he pulled her around to face him.

The blue lights of the aquarium tanks softened everything around them. No one else was on the dance floor, and even if there was, there was no way he could look away from the siren in front of him.

"Do you dance much?" Vi put his hand on her waist as they, or rather she, moved instinctively to the beat. He just did his best to follow the lead she was setting.

"No." He grinned as she wrapped her arms around his neck, her hips brushing against his. "All of my limited musical talents were on show when we sang the 'Monster Mash.'"

"Relax." She shifted in his arms.

He wasn't sure that was possible when the beauty before him was sending all sorts of thoughts through his mind with her movements.

She turned, so her butt was pressed against him, laughing as Fiona, Patrick and several other guests joined them on the floor. For the next twenty minutes, he lost track of everything except for the feel of her against him, the beat of the music and the happiness flowing through him.

"All right folks!" The DJ called out as the fast song softened into a slow ballad. "The bride and groom and all of the wedding party need to get going. Big day tomorrow and I will be here to rock these tunes. But let's set the right mood for the final dance."

A love song started to play. The couples around them pulled each other close. Beck didn't hesitate.

Vi's soft arms went around his neck. "Thank you for dancing with me." She sighed as she laid her head his shoulder.

He pressed his lips to the top of her head. "Of course."

"It was nice to have a dance partner." She kissed his cheek.

It was a sad statement but given that Thomas had not stepped onto the dance floor with his partner, it didn't surprise him. "I will be your dance partner anytime you want."

It was promise he wasn't really in a position to make. When they got back to Bangor…well, he'd love to keep seeing her. Explore more dates and such. But he wasn't a forever partner.

The music ended. The couples around them all clung to each other for a moment. He was glad, because it meant that it wasn't obvious to anyone, but him, that he didn't let her go the moment the music stopped.

"Guess it's time to get back on the bus and then grab some beauty rest." Violet pulled back but put her hand in his as they followed the rest of the crowd out.

"I had fun tonight, Vi. A lot of it."

"Even if my college bestie threatened you?" She giggled as they stepped onto the party bus.

"Fiona didn't threaten me—technically." She'd never actually uttered the threat.

Sliding onto the bench seat, Violet pulled him down next to her. "I think we both know not uttering it is more threatening."

True.

CHAPTER EIGHT

VIOLET PULLED HER shoes off as soon as she and Beck stepped into their hotel room. She stretched her toes. "I know they aren't everyone's favorite footwear, but I'll take the comfy orthopedic shoes I wear with my scrubs over heels every single day."

Perfection.

That was the best descriptor for tonight. That was something she hadn't counted on when she ran into Thomas and his new wife by the elevator. Beck was the best date she could ask for. He might not have many moves on the dance floor, but he'd stood with her. Loosening up his hips and swishing to the music.

She'd seen the photographer snap a few photos of them. She'd have to ask Fiona to send one or two. Maybe this wasn't forever, but she wanted to document it. She felt alive around Beck.

Thomas had refused to set foot on the dance floor. He said he had two left feet. Maybe he did, but she thought the real issue was that he didn't want people watching him do something he wasn't very good at.

His wife had dutifully stood by him tonight. Violet hadn't paid them much attention. She hoped Dove was happy, but she was glad it wasn't her sitting out of the dances anymore.

"Sit. I'll rub your feet." Beck took off his jacket and tie.

He unbuttoned the top two buttons of his dress shirt, and she bit back the groan coming up her throat. No man had ever looked as good as Beck did.

"I can't ask you to do that." She kissed his cheek. Why couldn't she stop touching him, even though the nearly platonic touch wasn't close to what her body craved?

They'd shared that one kiss after karaoke. One glorious kiss. Since then…disappointment. No. Touching him and being touched by him were never disappointing. Violet just wanted more.

She grabbed her sweatpants and an old T-shirt. "I'm going grab a quick shower." Maybe if she was in the decidedly unsexy outfit, it would keep her thoughts in control.

Pulling her wet hair into a loose braid for sleeping, she took a deep breath. Beck was sweet, fun to hang out with and the perfect wedding date.

He was also gorgeous and she wanted another kiss. And so much more. If he kissed like a god, how would he make love? Slow, sensuously. Taking all night to…

Heat flooded her entire body. The sweats and oversize shirt were doing nothing to chill her own need.

Straightening her shoulders, she tried to put the desire into a mental box. He'd mentioned dating—and then the shift from hell and exhaustion had ruined that. They were having a good time at a wedding. That was all.

Stepping out of the bathroom, she nearly fell over the scene he made on the bed. The only one bed in the room. He'd said he'd use the pullout couch, but she'd told him there was no reason they couldn't behave as adults and share.

Now, though, she wondered if she could make it.

Beck was in a tight white undershirt and loose blue sweatpants. He was reading a book, his glasses just a little lower on the edge of his nose. He looked like an underwear model.

Looking over the spine, he grinned, then set the book down. "Come here." He held up some of the lotion she'd brought with her.

"What?" Her mouth went dry as her mind started to spin fantasies.

"Your feet." Beck pointed. "I know a shower can help, but those shoes looked vicious and you have to be in them tomorrow too. So come on."

He patted the bed and her knees buckled. "Beck—"

"You aren't asking, I'm offering. Let me take care of you."

Take care of you.

When was the last time any man had taken care of her? She racked her brain but not a single instance ran through her head. Sure, there'd been times when she'd asked Thomas for help, or asked one of her other boyfriends for something, but they'd never actually taken care of her.

In fact, Thomas had made certain she never felt comfortable asking. A red flag she hoped he'd corrected before marrying his new wife.

"Thank you." She scooted onto the bed and put her feet over his lap. Even through the two layers of sweats between them, she could feel the heat of his body. Or maybe it was just her imagination playing through something so delicious.

Beck put some of the lotion on her feet. "Oh, this smells nice." He gripped her right foot, his fingers lying over the top as his thumbs pressed the bottom of her foot an inch or so beneath her toes.

"Ohhh." The sigh flew out of her mouth as his thumbs circled the pressure points. She'd meant to say something about that being her daily moisturizing lotion. It had a pleasant scent, but it wasn't a strong perfume. However, all the words fell from her brain as he touched her.

"Lean back."

The command was soft, but she was incapable of doing anything but following. "How did you get so good at this?"

Beck slid off the bed, pulling her feet with him so that they were at the edge of the bed, while he knelt on the floor.

"My mother. In her last few years, her feet hurt terribly from nerve pain, but she had dementia and couldn't remember any new people. She didn't remember me, either, or at least not that I was her son. But she knew that I was safe; so she let me rub her feet. It calmed her and made it a little easier for her to walk short distances."

She leaned up on her elbows looking over at him. "I bet she liked that."

He titled his head, but didn't look up from her feet, the pressure never stopping.

"She did. They had me late in life. The surprise baby. Dad had been gone for a year when she had to go into assisted living. I think of them often, and I bet they are having a blast together on the other side. Maybe even traveling to different parts of the universe."

That was such a nice thought. A tinge sad, but she could hear the happy memories even in his grief.

Violet hadn't had a close relationship with her parents. Her mother had filed the divorce papers the day after Violet moved out. Both parents seemed to blame her for how their lives had turned out. Or maybe she was just a reminder of the decades of life with a partner they'd hated.

If they'd asked, she'd have preferred two homes to the broken one she'd grown up in.

They fell into an oddly comforting silence.

"All right, my hands are aching. How are your feet?"

Oh. Violet sat up, stretched and wiggled her toes. "I feel great. I'm so sorry. I should have paid more attention to the time."

Beck waved his hand like he was brushing the apology away. "I'm fine." He grinned and headed into the bathroom.

She felt amazing. And she planned to return the favor.

When he came back out of the bathroom, he sat on the bed and she could smell the minty toothpaste.

"Let me have your hand." She didn't wait for him to say anything.

Pulling his left hand into hers, she lifted his palm and ran her thumb down the middle. Fiona had taken a course in medical massage in college. Her friend had focused on hands and shoulders, since that was where most people kept most of the tension.

"Ohhh. I'm not the only one with a secret skill." Beck groaned and held up his other palm as soon as she touched it.

"Well, you don't have to be in heels all day, but it will be a long day for you, too."

Beck wrapped his fingers around hers. "Vi." His blue gaze captured hers.

The hotel room was a decent size, but in this moment, it felt like there was nowhere to go to escape his jeweled eyes.

Like I want to go anywhere.

"Beck." His name tasted so good on her tongue. Before she could think of anything else, she leaned forward. Her lips brushed his and the world exploded.

Vi was kissing him. Really kissing him. For no reason. There was no one to impress in this room. No ex, so no need to make a point. No questions to avoid.

No learning moment or silly bet.

Just Beck and Vi.

Heaven.

That was what this hotel room was. A slice of perfection. Their slice of perfection.

His hands cupped her face, willing her to come a little closer. She scooted toward him, her legs wrapping around his waist.

Heaven.

"Beck." She kissed him again. Her hands circled his back as she fit against him.

The cotton shirt he wore was fire against his skin. Dear God he ached to pull it off. Take her shirt off and spend the evening losing himself in her body.

And he would too. There were no illusions here. Vi was the most beautiful, kind, sweet, funny woman he'd ever met. He'd accept any exhaustion in order to spend the next several hours worshiping her body.

But tomorrow was her friend's wedding. She was bridesmaid and had responsibilities from the moment breakfast ended to the end of the reception.

"Vi." He cupped the back of her neck. "Vi."

"You already said my name." She grinned, then kissed him again. The feel of her smile against his lips was a huge turn on.

"You have a big day tomorrow." He pulled back, feeling every bit of the playful pout she gave him.

Moving her hips against him, he had no doubt she knew how turned on he was. "It is going to be very busy indeed. All the more reason to release some tension tonight."

"Mmm." He raised a brow. "Taking care of your tension is not an issue." Beck slid his fingers down her back.

She tipped her head and dropped her hand to the bulge in his lap. "You are tense too."

He gripped her hand, pulling it to his lips, where he kissed each finger while holding her chocolate gaze. "I am. But the first time I sleep with you, I plan to make it last as long as possible."

Violet looked at him, then looked over her shoulder at the hotel clock on the nightstand. Recognition crossed her gaze. It was already so late.

"Tomorrow?"

"Mmm-hmm." Tomorrow. He'd get to spend the entire day planning out exactly how he wanted to make her come. Not a bad way to spend the day. The expectation alone would have them both in perfect sync.

"But for now." He put his hands around her back, leaning her against the pillows.

"Is this the part where you put me to bed? Not sure I can sleep quite yet." She grinned and kissed him, her teeth nipping at his bottom lip.

"Why don't you let me help with that?" Beck trailed kisses down her neck. "Untie your sweatpants, Vi."

She took a deep breath and followed the command.

Beck slipped his hand down her pants, stroking her through her silky panties. He craved her nakedness, but if he stripped her, the minute control he was maintaining on his own need would crack.

The little cries echoing from her lips were going to drive him mad in his dreams tonight. He teased her mouth with his tongue before slipping his hand into her panties.

"Beck." She arched against him as he pressed his thumb to her clit, circling the tiny bud, adjusting his pressure with each sigh he drew from her lips.

"Beck!"

The soft pant drew a moan from him. "Vi."

"I like you calling me Vi. No one else does." The words were broken with pants.

She was close, and he slipped a finger into her, his thumb never shifting its pressure. She broke as he stroked her core, his name on her lips as she crested the mountain.

Vi didn't break his gaze as he pulled his hand from her pants. Neither of them had discarded any clothes, but he'd never been more turned on.

Tomorrow.

"Think you can sleep tonight?" Beck slid onto the pillow beside her.

"Beck." His name was a sigh on her lips, the result of her orgasm and exhaustion. He pulled her into his arms.

"Good night, Vi." He kissed the top of her head, holding her tightly as her soft sighs disappeared as she drifted off to sleep.

Heaven.

Well rested did not even begin to describe her this morning. She'd slept like the dead, and awakened in Beck's arms. He'd snoozed beside her, but she was very aware of the erection pressing against her thigh.

Unfortunately there'd been no time for her to relieve his "tension." The bridal party and families were meeting for breakfast, then the bride and bridesmaids were headed to the suite Fiona had booked for the day for hair, makeup and bridal day fun.

"The buffet looks good." The words felt stilted after what they'd shared last night. What did one say in the morning after you'd had the best orgasm ever and never even dropped your drawers? Though his command to untie her pants had featured in several of her dreams she'd had last evening.

"It does. Are you hungry?" There was a hint of a sparkle in his eye.

She was ravenous. For food…and him.

Heat warmed her cheeks, and she had to look away from Beck's blue eyes. Seriously, if the flame went out on the heaters keeping the sausages warm, she was pretty sure her touch alone would reignite it.

They grabbed their food and headed to one of the open four-seat tables.

"Do you have plans while I'm spending the day getting all dolled up?" Violet asked the question just as Beck put a big bite of egg in his mouth.

"Sorry." She giggled.

"That was less than perfect timing." Beck grinned as he reached for his coffee. "I don't really have any plans. I'm going to ask the concierge what is around besides the Frost Museum of Science, since we are getting an up close and personal version of that for the wedding tonight."

"Text me any fun pictures." There wasn't time for her to have much of a tourist jaunt this time, but she hadn't lived and worked in this city in a decade so she wouldn't have been a helpful guide anyway.

"Of course."

"Violet." Thomas's tone broke through her morning joy and she didn't bother to smile as he and his wife set their food down at the two open chairs.

Surely the man didn't want to have breakfast with her and Beck. "Thomas, there are open seats—"

"These work fine." He pulled out a napkin and spread it across his lap. The people at the table next to them had turned their heads, and heat poured onto her cheeks. How many times had he made her feel uncomfortable before?

Countless.

And his poor wife. In the morning light, it was clear how much they looked alike. She didn't meet Violet's gaze as she stabbed a fork through the cut strawberry on her plate.

This was beyond awkward.

Beck caught her gaze and raised an eyebrow. If she wanted him to make a scene he would. But this was Fiona's wedding day. At least a handful of the people down here were wedding guests. If this became a hissy fit, and Thomas was not above that, then guests would gossip over it at the wedding. It was just human nature.

She was not going to be gossip—that was the entire reason Beck was here!

"I wanted to talk to you." Thomas cleared his throat, picked up his knife and fork but didn't cut his food.

Beck's right hand slid along her knee. At least she wasn't facing her ex and her look-a-like alone.

"We haven't seen each other or talked in years. I don't know what there is to discuss. We are just here to celebrate Fiona and Patrick." Violet laid her hand over Beck's, squeezing it once. With any luck Thomas would take the hint—for the first time in his life.

"I want the royalties for our book. All of them."

Direct had never been a problem for Thomas, but she hadn't even finished one cup of coffee. No workup to it. No beating around the bush.

"You aren't training dogs in Maine. This one told me that last night." Thomas pointed his still unused fork at Beck.

She hadn't trained dogs in Maine, hadn't thought of training them, until she'd met up with Beck at the Happy Feet Gym.

But even if she wasn't training them, she'd written the book. Sure, his name was on it, but all he'd contributed was gripes.

"Vi does train. I just didn't want to discuss it with you." Beck let out an overdramatic sigh. "She is my girlfriend, man. You left her at the altar. You don't get to know her present. Why can't you see that?"

Thomas blinked at Beck's rebuke.

Violet leaned over and kissed Beck's cheek. She laid a hand on the other side of his face. "Thank you."

"So you are training?"

"She is working with our intermediate team. The first session she had with us was life-changing."

"Beck." That was a bit of an overstatement. The one training session they'd had was good. And there'd been immediate improvements, but life-changing was not even close to a description she'd use.

"No. You are amazing. In fact with your training, I bet we place this year at regionals. A first for the gym." Beck's gaze was fully focused on her.

She could hear Thomas's huff, and she knew he could, too. But Beck never broke her gaze.

"Thank you."

"A small gym in Maine does not make you a full-time trainer. I could take you to court over the royalties. Make it clear to them that I'm the real brains behind the book and that I only let you get your name on it because we were, ahem, involved at the time." That was an empty threat.

They'd signed a contract with the publishing house who'd insisted they have separate contracts since they weren't legally married. A small grace that she hadn't been grateful for at the time. She'd had a lawyer look at it after Thomas left, just in case he pulled this kind of stunt.

It had taken longer than she'd expected, but there was no way for him to sue for such a thing. And if he did, he'd lose and have to pay her court fees. But…

"You never gave my grandmother's tablecloth back. What on earth makes you think I'd be willing to do a single thing for you." She crossed her arms. Nana had cross-stitched the little gingerbread family and Christmas trees and given it to Violet as an engagement gift. The fact that Thomas had taken it and refused to even acknowledge he had it when she'd texted him repeatedly was low enough. The idea that he and his family were using it, a gift for her, from her nana, a woman who hadn't lived to see him leave her at the altar.

A small blessing, for her nana would have hunted him down.

"I don't have the tablecloth."

"You do." She grabbed her phone, opened the pictures and spun it toward him. "I snapped that pic of your table when Fiona reposted a picture of the tablecloth that your mother took last Christmas."

She saw Dove's eye widen, but Thomas's wife didn't add anything to the conversation. That was fine. This wasn't her fight.

Thomas looked at the photo, let out a sigh, then lifted the coffee cup to his lips. He took a long sip, his eyes never leaving her face. Once that stare might have made her stand down. Now all it did was make her straighten her back and raise her chin.

"That isn't your tablecloth. And we are discussing the book." A book that at this point wasn't bringing in many royalties. Maybe it was time for another—without Thomas's name on it.

The thought punched through her brain. Another…

There was so much she'd left out of the first book. Trainer's Guide Version Two had been her pretend nickname for an idea she'd let die when Thomas walked out of her life. Another thing she'd let him steal.

"I guess this conversation is over. See you in Boston for the regionals—with your team." Thomas pushed back from the table.

"Just so you know." Beck leaned forward, and she saw Thomas startle just a little. "As a show of goodwill you should give that tablecloth back. It would be a shame if news like that went viral in social media posts. I'm sure everyone who frequents your gym and still has great memories of Violet would be shocked to learn you took that."

"Who says they have great memories?"

Vi tilted her head, imagining her fingers wrapping around his stupid little neck.

"Of course they have great memories of Vi. She is the best." Beck put an arm around her shoulders, and all the murderous thoughts evaporated as he planted his lips on hers.

Beck was staking a claim. Letting Thomas know that he was no longer important in her life. Usually Violet hated that kind of male protection, but with Beck, part of her wished it was real.

CHAPTER NINE

"WHERE DID YOU learn to dance?" Beck wasn't ashamed to admit that there was no way to keep up with Vi on the dance floor. Luckily, she didn't seem bothered by his awkward movements.

And she had an innate ability to dodge his feet if they strayed too close to her toes.

Vi let out a giggle as she twirled through his arms with the fast beat. "I signed up for class by mistake."

The song ended and the DJ started a ballad. Finally. Pulling Violet into his arms was a lovely, but it also let him catch his breath. They'd been on the dance floor since the bride and groom opened it with their first dance. And he suspected they'd close it down.

Which was fine with him.

"How does one sign up for a dance class by mistake?" He'd taken dozens of classes over time. More extreme ones after his parents passed. Skydiving certifications, deep-sea diving, hang gliding…anything that sparked his interest and got his blood pumping. But never by mistake.

Violet laid her head against his shoulder. There were others on the dance floor, but they evaporated as he kissed her and spun her slowly around the floor.

"I filled out paperwork at the little hobby shop in my hometown. They had all sorts of things and I spent most of my childhood summers there. I meant to sign up for the stained-glass crafting course, but I transposed the numbers and ended up in beginning jazz. I *was not* dressed correctly for that first class let me tell you."

"I bet." Beck pulled her even closer, letting his finger run down her back. The navy bridesmaid dress had a classic, modest, scoop neck. But the back had nearly sent him to his knees when he watched her walk down the aisle.

The deep vee opened nearly to the top of her perfect ass. There was no way she was wearing more than pasties over her taut breasts. A single pearl drop necklace hung down the middle of her back. It was formal and sexy as hell. "Never did learn how to craft stained glass. I did take every dance class I could fit in my schedule. In fact, I took so many in college I actually earned a double major in biology and dance."

"Have you taken any classes at Spotlight Studios?" He didn't know much about dance classes, but he'd been to more than one recital. A few years ago his friend Marcus's little boy had signed up for tap. He had almost backed out of the recital because he'd been made fun of in school. Marcus had called on all his friends to sit in the front row and cheer him on.

Last year his son had started modern dance, and the whole cheering section was right in place to cheer him on. It was fun. When it was time for the spring recital, he'd have to make sure to invite Violet. She'd love it.

His feet stumbled, and Vi grabbed his shoulders.

"Careful there!" She kissed his cheek.

"Sorry." It was weird to be glad that he'd nearly smashed her toes several times tonight. But it meant that Violet wouldn't think this was anything more than a rhythm misstep rather than his heart breaking a little.

He didn't know what this fling would look like, but he

doubted it included bringing Vi to a yearly event—even one he knew she'd love. It hurt to think that she wouldn't be next to him.

That was a problem for future Beck. The list of things his future self would have to deal with was adding up, but he wasn't going to think of them.

Right now he was focusing on the woman in front of him. On the woman coming alive before him.

"Since I nearly mashed your toes, you didn't answer. Have you taken any dance classes since you moved to Bangor?"

She stiffened in his arms and the song changed before she answered. She bolted from his arms without a word. Not that he really needed a verbal answer.

The Violet he'd known for the past few years and the woman who'd been dancing in his arms were two different creatures. Both were magnificent. But he couldn't help but feel like the Violet currently holding the bride's hips as they started a conga line was the real version.

Would she stay this person when they returned to Bangor? Or would she put this form of herself back into hibernation? As the conga line stretched around the room, he joined in, enjoying the smile Vi passed back as the giant snake of wedding guests enjoyed the silly dance.

"Now that that has ended…" the DJ said as Violet found her way back to Beck.

"I could use a glass of water." She wrapped an arm around his waist.

"I'm parched." Beck brushed her lips with his as they turned to head off the dance floor.

They hadn't taken two steps when the DJ continued. "Time for all the unmarried ladies to make their way to the dance floor. It's bouquet toss time, and Fiona has a twist for it."

"Of course she does." Violet giggled as Fiona moved onto the dance floor carrying her bouquet with at least a dozen ribbons attached to it.

"Come on, single ladies! I know who all of you are, and I have a ribbon for each of you *with* your name on it! You are not getting out of my game!"

Violet shook her head as Fiona made direct eye contact with her.

"I think that last part was a dig at you." Beck tapped her hip with his and kissed the top of her head. "Go. I'll have refreshments ready as soon as you step off the floor."

"If she wasn't the bride..." Violet kissed him, then made her way to the group, grabbing the lone ribbon on the floor.

Fiona told the women they were doing a bridal maypole and when she cut their ribbon they were out. Then she pulled a sleep mask over her eyes, raised the bouquet above her head and the music started.

Fiona seemed to take her time using the scissors, though maybe it was harder to cut ribbon blindfolded than she'd counted on.

Thomas sidled up to Beck, who grimaced. What had Violet ever seen in this awful man?

"You know this is what she wants, right? Better hope Violet doesn't get that bouquet if you aren't ready to pop the question."

Beck did not bother to address that ridiculous statement.

Unfortunately his silence didn't seem to be a deterrent for Thomas. "For as long as I knew Violet, she talked of getting married. Having a happy life with a partner. Nights in and all that jazz." Thomas crossed his arms as he stood next to Beck, his gaze focused on the single ladies in the center.

One lady in particular.

"Do you have a point? Or are you just not over her? I get it. She is remarkable. I'd hate losing that." His mouth suddenly dried as he realized he'd lose it too.

They were faking that they'd been together six months for the wedding—not that anyone had asked more than a handful of questions about how they met before moving onto other topics.

Thomas bristled and let out a low grunt. "I did not lose her. I was the one who ended things. Because I didn't want to be tied down."

Beck did not bother to argue that he was married now. To a woman who had to be questioning why her husband had an ex-fiancée who could be mistaken for her.

"Whoever is lucky enough to spend their life with Vi will never describe it as tied down." Jealousy flashed across his brain. Whoever that faceless person was would be forever lucky to have her by their side.

Getting to wake up next to her. Joke with her. Dance with her. That life was not going to be his. He wasn't ready to be married.

And Vi hadn't mentioned marriage.

Why would she?

Fiona cut the last string—Vi's string. For a moment he saw her face falter. She'd wanted the bouquet.

The moment was over before anyone else probably even noticed. She rolled up her ribbon and danced over to the woman now holding a miniature of Fiona's bouquet. She was laughing, all smiles. No hint of jealousy.

No doubt she was happy for her friend. But Thomas was right. Vi wanted marriage. She wanted to be the one tossing the bouquet or cutting the ribbon or whatever.

That wasn't a life he was ready for. Wasn't a life he was even sure he wanted.

We are having a fling. I shouldn't care that she wants more at some point in the future. With someone else.

Vi knew where they stood. This was fun. So why the hell did watching her dance with her ribbon above her head as the winner passed the bouquet around make him feel so empty?

Violet was exhausted. Fiona and Patrick's day had been perfect. That was what mattered. Right now she wanted exactly three things:

1. Kick off her high heels.
2. A shower.
3. Beck.

Pretty much in that order. Though she wouldn't mind joining number two and three together. As they got to the hotel door, she didn't bother to wait to start on number one, yanking the shoes off before Beck swung the door open.

"How are your feet?" Beck looked down at the toes that had been pinched most of the day and were certainly less than pretty at the moment.

Not where she wanted his focus.

"Sore." There was no point in fibbing. "But they will be fine. I'm going to grab a shower." She hesitated, then just decided to go for it. "Want to join me?"

Beck dropped his tux coat on the chair and pulled at the black tie he'd loosened in the elevator. "There isn't a lot of room in that shower." His voice was low. Husky.

Her body heated as she stepped toward him.

"I promise not to steal all the hot water, if that is what you are concerned about."

The grin spread across his face, and the dimples she was

so fond of appeared. "I'm starting the water." She turned and had to breathe deeply so that she didn't run to the bathroom.

Not that she wanted to flee. No. What she wanted was to take that sexy man, push him to the bed and have her way with him. Something she very much planned to accomplish after the day's makeup, hairspray and sweat were wiped from her body.

She started the water and felt his hands skim her back.

"I don't know if you picked this dress or if Fiona chose it, but Vi—it's the sexiest thing I've ever seen." His hands danced across the top of her ass, just below the cut of the dress.

"Fiona let us choose. They just all had to be navy. I will admit, since I ordered it online with just my measurements at the shop, I was more than a little stunned at how low the back cut was."

Fiona had screamed when she saw it during the try on when it was delivered to Violet's local dress shop from the Miami shop she'd ordered it from. If Fiona had been there in person instead of on a video call, she might have blown Violet's eardrums out. Fiona had clapped as she did a happy dance, then immediately suggested a statement back necklace. If there was one thing you could count on with Fiona as your friend, it was that she was going to root for you no matter what.

"This dress is going to feature in so many of my dreams." Beck's lips pressed against her shoulder as his hand traveled up her back then lowered again.

Violet turned and his hands cupped her butt, pulling her close.

"I need to pull the pins out of my hair so I can wash the hairspray out." She kissed his cheek and stepped to the mirror. The shower wasn't huge, but the bathroom was a very nice size overall.

Beck's hands strayed from her ass and he pulled one hair-pin, then another and another from her dark locks. His fingers gently rubbing her scalp as his mouth trailed kisses down her neck. Was there nothing this man wasn't good at?

Commitment.

Her brain supplied the answer without prompting, but Violet forced it away. She wasn't looking for commitment. She was looking for a fun time with a sexy man who wanted her. And Beck fit all of those criteria.

"I think I got all of them." Beck breathed the words against her ear as his hand cupped the back of her neck.

"Thank you." The words were thick. Every part of her body was alive, and he'd barely touched her.

"Take your dress off, Vi."

The command rocketed through her system. All she could do was obey. All she wanted to do was obey.

The straps of her dress slid down her arms, her body operating on pure desire as she stared at him. Steam swirled around them.

He unbuttoned his shirt and tossed it to the floor.

Her hands dragged along his abs, and she let out a soft sigh. Of course he looked even better shirtless.

Beck hooked a finger into the navy panties she'd bought for the day. The lacy undergarment was at her feet in seconds and the only thing standing between her and nakedness was the pasties she'd worn.

"I knew you were only in pasties." His thumb circled the silicone patch.

"Can't exactly wear a bra with that dress." Violet nipped his lip as she reached for the button of his tux pants. She was basically naked, and she wanted him wearing nothing at all too.

His pants lowered to the floor and she felt him step out

of them, but his mouth never left hers. "Come on. Into the shower." He turned her, his hand giving her ass the slightest push.

"The pasties."

"Will come off easier in the water." His lips trailed along her shoulder blade. "I plan to spend the entire night worshiping your body. I don't want anything sore."

His touch was electric, his kisses sublime. But it was the care he was showing on such a simple thing. The pasties had been on for more than eight hours and stayed on through the wedding and an evening of dancing.

She stepped into the shower. The hot water hit her back and she ached to stay under it, but she moved to let Beck stand in the water. The few times she'd showered with Thomas he'd insisted on standing in the water.

Beck gently grabbed her hips and pulled her into the water.

"You'll get cold." Her words were soft as his fingers stroked up her stomach then lower but never to where she ached for him most.

"*I* will be fine. You are the one who had a long day. I got to roam Miami, checking out anything I fancied, then spend the night dancing with the most interesting woman in the whole city." Beck reached for the soap, worked a lather up in his hands then started working his way along her body.

"Mmm." Violet leaned her head back. The heat of the shower and his touch melted together in a delicious manner there were no descriptors for.

His hands circled her breasts, soap and warm water making quick work of the pasties. Then his thumbs were circling her nipples.

"Beck…"

"Turn around, Vi."

She was putty in his hands. She turned on command, very aware of the thick rod against her butt. Violet wiggled her ass against it, enjoying the hiss of breath as he tried to stay focused on her.

He poured a little shampoo into his hands, then started working it through her hair. "Mmm."

"I like it when I steal all the words from you." Beck kissed the soft skin behind her ears as he washed her hair.

She thrust her back against his length and he made the same little hiss as he rushed the air out. "And *I* enjoy making you do that."

He turned her to allow the water to start rinsing the shampoo from her locks. When it was gone, she grabbed the conditioner, finished up her hair routine, then pulled him into the water.

Last night he'd touched her. Brought her to completion with no demand for his own need. Tonight...tonight she was going to touch him. She soaped up her hands, then let herself explore Beck with the same enthusiasm he'd done to her.

As she wrapped her hands around his length, he let out a groan. "Vi."

The nickname on his lips as she stroked him was such a turn on.

His hand slipped between her legs, finally gliding over the sensitive spot she craved. It vanished so fast as he turned the water off.

"If we stand in here in any longer, I'm going to lose myself, Vi." He grabbed a towel from the rack and wrapped her in it, before grabbing another and drying himself faster than she thought possible.

I guess anything is possible when you're motivated.

She stepped out of the shower. Steam filled the whole room.

Beck followed her, grabbing a spare towel to pull the excess moisture from her hair.

"Beck." The care was lovely, and excruciating.

"I want you, Vi. I want you more than I've ever wanted anyone or anything." Beck's lips lingered on hers as he dropped the towel to the floor, then reached for the one wrapped around her body.

He pulled it away, reached for the bathroom door, then gathered her into his arms.

There was nothing Beck wanted more than to bury himself in Violet and lose himself in the sensation. But he'd sworn that during their first time together he was going to worship her. And there was so much of her left to adore.

Carrying her to the bed, he laid her gently on the edge, then he spread her legs and licked her core. He'd longed to do this last night.

Strip her. Taste her. Lose himself in the perfection of Vi.

"Beck."

His name on her lovely lips made him harder—something that shouldn't have been possible.

Slipping his hands under her butt, he pulled her even closer, drinking her in. Her legs wrapped around his head, urging him more as her fingers wrapped in his hair. She was panting, her hips bucking as his tongue darted around her clit.

"Beck!" She moaned his name, but this time as he felt her crest over the edge. He pulled one hand from under her and grabbed the condom he'd laid out on top of the nightstand this morning.

He didn't stop kissing her as he pulled the sheath from its wrapping and slid it down his length.

"Beck. Seriously. I need you. Now. Now."

He grinned against her thigh as trailed a line of kisses there. "I like it when you demand that."

Beck slipped between her legs, pushing himself in just a little and sucking in a deep breath.

"No teasing. Please, please." Violet wrapped her legs around his hips, pulling him deeper.

His fingers moved through her hair as his lips caught hers. "Not teasing. Just trying to keep from losing myself so completely in a second."

Violet claimed his mouth as he filled her.

Once joined, their bodies moved as one, their breathing seeming to synchronize as she climaxed again. Finally he let himself experience the same release.

CHAPTER TEN

"NICE WORK!" Violet clapped as Tim and Pickle did a perfect 270-degree transition and raced onto the A-frame then across the finish line.

Beck and Toaster were at the starting line; Beck celebrating, Toaster looking at the course, ready for her turn. That dog lived for agility.

Since returning from Miami last week, she and Bear had spent a few days at Beck's after shift. The two of them had agreed when the fling started that it went on for as long as they both wanted it. And that no one was getting down on one knee.

It was easy with Beck. There were no expectations—just fun. It was nice. But there was a heaviness that she couldn't always force away.

This was the life she'd planned. Working as a vet, running an agility team and coming home to a partner who made her feel like she was the best catch in the world. For years she'd put that life away. Refused to acknowledge the dream she'd held for so long. Now she had part of it.

As she watched Beck start Toaster off on the course, she swallowed the small lump in the back of her throat. They were having fun. He wasn't a forever partner, but that was all right, for now.

"Good job, Toaster." Beck laughed as the dog jumped into his arms at the end of the course.

"It was a good run," Violet said as she joined them.

"But?" Beck raised an eyebrow.

"But, Toaster is still not comfortable with the blind approaches." The dog was hesitating on obstacles that were not clear from the dismount from the last obstacle. It was a common issue.

Dogs wanted to see their whole path. They wanted to know what was coming. It was a natural response that could cost points in a competition.

A competition she wanted this team to place in. Thomas was going to be there, and he was going to judge how they did. Kicking his ass would be such a great way to put the final nail in the coffin of her past.

She should have told him to stick it when he asked for the royalties of the book. Having that much audacity was a skill— one that she hated to admit had gotten him access to places he really had no business being.

A mediocre man riding the coattails of others did not deserve anything. Unfortunately she knew he was petty enough to refuse to return the tablecloth…or even destroy it. Having it was his cruel reminder to her that he'd taken something she couldn't replace.

"Toaster has always struggled with blind approaches." Beck passed his dog a training treat, rewarding her for the good run. And it had been a good run—just not great.

"Well, we have a couple more weeks before regionals in Boston. So we will focus on everyone's main issues. Toaster doesn't like blind obstacles, Posy is not a fan of the collapsed tunnel, Tuna had multiple contact faults tonight where she didn't touch the obstacle the right way and Pickle barely got over the bar."

"Barely." Tim smiled. "But she cleared it and that means no dropped bar fault."

"Her back legs were millimeters from it, Tim. If she is nervous at competition, which is always possible, those millimeters will be an easy slip for her." She'd told the team about her ex. About how she'd love for the Happy Feet Gym to crush the fancy gym she'd used to work at. They'd all rally around to do their best to place.

Which she was grateful for. But it meant they were going to have to work harder than anyone but Nancy had worked at Happy Feet. Tonight was their first full workout. The first real test.

"Okay, but I mean, she cleared it. I get what you are saying but," he said, shrugging, "I don't get why we are focusing on a dropped bar that didn't drop."

She looked at the group and their dogs. "I know this is hard." Maybe this was too much all at once. It was a lot to ask a team that usually used the trip as a fun excuse to get out of town for the weekend. But they were already so close. With just a bit of work they could clear the hurdles—literally and figuratively.

"Things that are worthwhile generally are." Beck nodded to her.

She gave him a quick smile. On the few occasions that Thomas had been on the gym floor with her, he'd vanished when even the smallest bit of conflict had arisen.

"They are." Violet took a deep breath. "If you have changed your minds and do not wish to aim for medals, that's fine. But we make that decision tonight. As a group. One person wants out, then we go to Boston for fun only. No pressure."

"What about your ex?" Grace covered her heart with her hand. "I mean come on. That guy sounds like he needs to be taken down at least one peg."

Grace had an ex-husband who was a real piece of work according to Beck. She was living a little vicariously through Vi's desire to stick it to Thomas. It was sweet, but this was a team effort.

"I appreciate the support. But this is your team. I am an interloper and asking a lot."

"You are our coach." Lisa crossed her arms. "*Not* an interloper. Assuming you want to be our coach. I mean I know you are just getting back into agility and you have the vet clinic and Beck…dear God someone else say something so I can stop blathering."

Beck reached down and gave Toaster a rub behind her floppy ears. "You know I am in."

"Tim." Grace turned her focus on him and the others followed.

"Nope. Nope, we aren't ganging up on Tim." Violet stepped forward. "He gets to make his own decision."

"I choose the team and trying to medal. I'm sorry about the question."

"Don't apologize for questions." Violet had always had an open forum with her clients. She knew agility. Knew dogs. Knew competitions.

She knew coaches who felt that because they knew those things, it wasn't a client's position to question the coach. She felt no need to gatekeep the information.

"You asked why millimeters matter. The truth is that they may not, but if Pickle is tired before running the course from excitement, or nerves, or something she can't tell us about because she is a dog and we do not speak the same language then it might matter." Violet made a cute face at the dog as Pickle tilted her head as though she was absorbing everything from this very important conversation.

"If she is used to being just millimeters above the bar, then there is no room for error." Tim nodded. "Makes sense."

"It does." She put her hand out, palm down. The others followed suit, laying one hand on top of the other. "On three we yell team."

"One," Violet said as she looked to Grace.

"Two." Grace nodded at Beck.

"Three!" he roared.

"Team!" The cheer went up and the dogs all turned and looked at their humans like they'd lost their minds. But none of them barked or got excited.

That was good. Because the competition would be wild even though the dogs in attendance would be well behaved. Spectator noise. Scents galore. Excitement. It was a recipe for doggies to lose control.

"Nice work tonight. See everyone in two days." She waved to the group as Tim, Lisa and Grace gathered their pups and headed off.

"You are amazing. Do you know that?" Beck wrapped his arms around her. "You handled Tim with such skill."

"I was just answering his questions, Beck. Nothing special." She kissed his cheek, enjoying the feel of his arms wrapped around her.

He squeezed her and stepped back. "Why don't we grab Bear and let them play in the course for a little while. See if we can get Toaster a little more comfortable with blind approaches and get a little exercise for Bear."

"Hey." Violet playfully punched his shoulder. "Bear ran

around a few times, and he went for a walk today. That is a lot of work for him."

"Uh-huh." Beck shook his head as he walked back out onto the course.

She went over to where Bear was sleeping. It wouldn't hurt for him to run a few more laps. The pittie would never be an agility competition dog, but he was a good boy.

"Come on, honey, let's go get a little exercise."

"Sorry we are just having a slow night." Beck slid onto the couch where Vi was already starting to pull up the streaming services.

"No need to apologize." She crossed her legs, putting the bowl of popcorn she'd popped in the center.

Tonight was supposed to be a fun date. He'd had the best plan. But at the last minute the surprise had to be rescheduled. It was perfect too. So much better than movies on the couch. A mini adventure right in town.

"I swear I had an idea." He'd talked it up too. Made such a big deal out of it. And now she was eating popcorn on his couch looking through horror flick choices.

Violet tilted her head as she met his gaze. "Beck, I wanted to hang out tonight. I was excited for the surprise, and I will be excited when it happens. But that does not mean that a night rummaging through the solid campy horror flicks you have available on your streaming services is not just as exciting. I like hanging out at home and relaxing just us."

Hanging out at home—his parents' favorite thing. It was nice. Better than nice. He could almost see why his parents gave up their adventures. *Almost.*

"Horror movies. I would have thought you were into rom-coms." She loved the idea of love—that was clear in the instant Fiona cut Vi's ribbon.

The woman who'd showed up in Miami for the wedding had come home to Maine. Vi didn't just go to work, go home and repeat the process. That was good, but he kept wondering when she might decide to end this fling and find the man who'd get down on one knee. The one who'd let her toss the bouquet and dance with her in an elegant white gown.

He hated that future man.

"I like rom-coms too. But there is something about silly horror flicks. The campy ones that are working too hard and have low budgets so obvious it's funny. Or the ones that follow the exact script of the one survivor—always a teen girl who is very into her virginity."

Beck didn't have much knowledge on the genre. "I don't know that I have ever watched a horror flick."

Popcorn teetered on the edge of the bowl but somehow managed not to spill over as Violet turned toward him. "How! How, as a teen boy, did you not watch any of the *Friday the 13th* movies, or *Zombieland* or *Freddy vs Jason* or *Predator* or—"

"Whoa!" Beck held up his hands as well-known but, at least for him, unwatched franchises rattled out of Vi's mouth. "I know those movies but, if you keep listing flicks, I'm going to lose track fast."

Vi scooted a little closer to him on the couch. "Sorry, but I thought it was a staple of teen male experience to watch gory movies. Or at least to take girls to horror movies in the hopes that they would lean super close to you and snuggle during the whole movie."

He'd had some male friends who'd certainly used that

dating route but not him. "My parents didn't think they were appropriate."

"I can see that. Nightmares and all."

"That is a reason most would use, but my mom thought that they leaned into stereotypes and focused too much on using sex as a weapon for murder. She is credited on one of dad's anthropology papers about how the roles ancient societies placed on purity can be seen in modern movie franchises."

"Wow." Vi's eyes were huge as she turned to look at the list of movies pulled up on the screen. "I bet that was an interesting paper."

"It was well received by my father's colleagues." He remembered them poring over papers, talking excitedly with each other. The papers seemed to be all over the house that year rather than confined to their study as they usually were.

"I still have it on the shelf in their study. That room is mostly the same as it was." It was their happy place. And he'd loved to admit that was the reason he couldn't change it. That would be the selfless reason. A son still tied to his lost parents.

But the truth was that it was his reminder room. His dad's desk, with the image of their wedding day and a garden tea party. His father's favorite pictures. The ones showing the "boring" life he was so proud of. Beck used it as a reminder not to get stuck under papers, under matrimony—at least not for a while.

None of that was happy date night stuff, though. And on a night where they were already doing something less than thrilling, he wasn't going to think about the static life his parents had lived here. "Did a boy take you to a horror movie and wrap his arms around you when you got scared? Is that why you like them so much?"

Vi laughed, but it held very little humor. "No. I started

watching them long before I was allowed to date. My mom hated them. I mean like refused to be in the house when they were on. So whenever she and Dad were having a blowout, he'd pop one on in the living room, sit on the couch and wait for her to leave."

Beck wasn't sure what to say. There were thousands of ways to get into the genre, and he'd have guessed all of them before that. "So you and your dad watched the movies together?" It seemed like a weird way to bond with a parent.

"Oh no. Dad didn't watch them. He just started them so she would leave." Vi let out a sigh. "Neither were good communicators. But hey, at least I know pretty much every horror flick available in the last thirty years."

"Yeah. That is a bonus." Beck wasn't sure what to say to that. He could count on one hand the number of times he'd seen his parents fight. Oh sure, they disagreed, decently often even, but they'd talked and worked it out.

Fights, the ones that resulted in a few days of hurt feelings, were so far removed from his youthful experience.

"So let's see, if you have never seen a horror movie, what do we start with? *Friday the 13th* is very well-known, but given the original release date of the first flick, it hasn't aged well. *Chucky* movies are another option."

"What is your favorite? That seems like the perfect place to start." He knew nothing more than the general themes of each. He remembered a few of his friends talking about the *Saw* franchise when it came out. Mostly because of the murderer's creepy mask.

"I am partial to zombie flicks. So we will grab one of those...after." She grabbed the popcorn bowl, stood and walked over to put it on the mantel. "I want to believe in our little angels." She looked over to the beds where Toaster and

Bear were currently resting—both sets of eyes focused on the popcorn bowl. "But I think leaving a bowl of popcorn out is a little too much temptation."

"Where are we going?" Beck stood.

"The study. I need to read that paper." She clapped. "I mean I'll never get to meet your parents. This seems like a fun get-to-know-you thing, plus anthropology and horror movies. I mean who wouldn't want to read that!"

Me.

He loved his parents. Missed them inordinately but their papers, the study, it was a reminder of all that they'd given up.

His mother had planned to get a PhD in women's studies— yes, she'd had a successful career as a civil engineer—but she'd never gone back to school. Something she'd talked about a lot in her dementia haze the last year. Hell, he'd even found her "filling out the paperwork" once on random sheets of paper in the long-term care facility.

His dad had gone on at least four trips a year before meeting his mother. He'd been fascinated by the motifs from the ancient world still driving modern ways. Threads of life and time he'd called it. Once he married his mother, the trips had gone from four, to one to none, so fast.

Still, it wouldn't take long to get the report and then see what Vi loved about zombie movies. And if she was happy, then so was he.

"Oh my gosh." Vi stepped into the study and he followed her.

The room still had the soft scent of his father's cologne. It wafted with the smell of paper and time. If Beck closed his eyes, he could see his father sitting in the chair, pointing out something to his mother, hugging her as she leaned into him.

They were like one. The years she'd spent on this side of the mortal coil without him had been the hardest. The dementia had stolen her memories of his death, but not the memory of their love. She looked for him until the day she joined him.

"Is this them?" She picked up the image from the desk. "I mean of course it is. You look just like your dad."

"I call that the boring picture." He grinned as he stepped toward her.

"Boring?" She ran a finger over the edge of the frame. "This isn't boring."

"It's a garden party, Vi." He looked at the image. His mom was holding a drink in her left hand, his father's hand in her right. He was looking at her as though there were no other partygoers while she talked to guests the camera captured in shadows on the ground only.

She looked at the photo one more time. "I guess we have different definitions of boring." She kissed his cheek and set the photo back down.

Beck swallowed the pain that truth sent through him. They had very different definitions of boring. Maybe one day settling down, giving up opportunities for traveling and excitement would seem better.

Hell, part of his brain had started whispering the second they'd turned the fake dating into an actual fling that this could be more. He'd fully accepted that this fling's timeline was in Vi's court. He'd stay as long as she wanted…but when she was ready to start the life she clearly still wanted, he'd step aside.

"Did your dad publish all these?" She looked at the bookcase, filled with Dr. Forester's name.

"Yes. Though most of them have his students listed as the primary author. After Dad made tenure, he used his name and support to help junior researchers get published but refused to take credit as the lead author." Beck ran his fingers over the books. It was one of his father's crowning achievements.

He'd often wondered if he'd seen his students as surrogate children. Probably.

"They sound lovely."

"They were." Beck looked around the room, his eyes falling on Vi. They'd have liked her.

No.

They'd have loved her. His father would have started talking about how he loved his "boring" life. His mother would have offered her engagement ring. A family heirloom passed on by her grandmother. One he still had upstairs, not that he planned to give it to anyone.

They'd have seen the spark that Vi brought to everything.

"Here is the paper." He grabbed it, eager to leave this room. The memories here were sweet, a little sad, but they were dangerously close to making him want the boring life. Movies, a standard spaghetti night—Thursdays, matching holiday pjs. A settled life.

There was nothing wrong with that. It just wasn't what he planned…at least not yet.

"Wonderful. I'll get it back to you as soon as I'm through." Vi grabbed his hand. "Now…the zombies."

She held up her free hand, opening and closing her mouth and crossing her eyes.

He chuckled at the ridiculous scene. "Is that what zombies act like?"

Violet shook her head, a playful frown pulling at her perfect lips. "The fact that you even have to ask that." She kissed his cheek. "Let the horror movie education begin!"

CHAPTER ELEVEN

"SO I WAS thinking the next time we have a down night, maybe we try *28 Days Later*. It's nearly thirty years old, but the zombies are fast and don't live forever." Beck winked before he headed into the on-call suite where a patient with a dog who they thought might have eaten a sock was waiting for an X-ray.

"Zombie movies. Not my thing." Lacey shook her head as she filled up her coffee mug and headed back out to the reception desk.

Violet liked zombie movies, and she was enjoying the fact that Beck apparently *really* liked zombie movies. It should be an exciting moment. Something for them to bond over.

So why did he keep insinuating that movie nights were down nights or boring? He'd apologized so many times for the movie night they'd had at his place three days ago. She wasn't sure what exciting event he'd had planned, but she knew it wasn't watching movies with a lap full of popcorn.

And then there'd been the picture of his parents. "The boring one" as he termed it. What she'd seen was happiness, love, life all wrapped into one photo. She knew why it held the place of honor on his father's desk.

Yes, the pictures of him in the Andes Mountains were exquisite and the image of his mother backpacking through Italy was gorgeous, but they didn't have the same life to them. The garden party perfectly captured two people, who according to Beck, had loved each other until the day they died.

If the universe was fair, they'd found each other on the other side and continued their journey together.

That was a kind of love her parents had never had. A kind of love she'd yearned for her whole life. That yearning had led her to nearly walk down the aisle to the wrong man. And then she'd spent ten years worrying it simply didn't exist.

But it did. People found it. People clung to it. How could Beck think that was boring?

It didn't matter. This was a fling. They were having fun.

Why do I have to keep reminding myself of that?

"Vi, the X-ray shows something in Roxy's large intestine." Beck walked to the screen in the back of the clinic, pushed a few things on the tablet and pulled up the image.

The sock was clear on the screen. Along with at least two others.

Crossing her arms, she blew out a breath. She'd hoped to prescribe some laxatives to the golden doodle if the X-ray showed a blockage. It wasn't uncommon for dogs to eat things they shouldn't—and it was a breed trait in goldendoodles.

Passing one sock might be possible, though there was never a guarantee. Passing three or more, would not be happening.

"How are the rest of her stats?" Maybe they could put off surgery until it was a standard business operating time. The procedure would still be expensive, but it would cut at least a thousand dollars off the bill.

"Not great. She's restless, and I had to muzzle her to do the exam. Roxy is dehydrated and no longer eating." Beck looked at his watch.

He was thinking the same thing she was. Roxy's owner, Marcy, loved her animal but for at least three socks, two hours on anesthesia and the emergency surcharge, it was going to be nearly five thousand dollars. Not a small price tag for anyone but a giant one for Marcy.

The woman had taken on the doodle after her sister had tired of the dog. A sweet and honorable decision. But, while all dogs were work, doodles required grooming, exercise to wear out their exuberant personalities and constant vigilance to keep them from doing things like attempting to digest socks.

Marcy did her best but tonight was going to be rough.

"All right. Let's go discuss options." She took one more look at the scan, then followed Beck to check on Roxy.

The dog was muzzled and lying against Marcy. Even without the X-ray the bulge in the lower belly was clear.

"I kept yelling at Trevor to pick up his damn socks. I told the bastard to pack his things while I'm here. It's one thing to ignore all the household chores while focusing on making your hacky sack YouTube videos, refuse to do a damn thing to help out with bills but to forget socks so Roxy gets sick. There is only so much I can take." Marcy buried her head in Roxy's ears, tears running down her face.

Beck looked at her, his wide eyes saying the same thing she was thinking. The first things Marcy listed were not small items in Violet's opinion. In fact they were giant red flags that should be relationship enders all on their own.

But since she'd overlooked all of Thomas's faults until it was literally impossible to do anything but acknowledge them, there was no way she was passing judgment of any kind here.

"Roxy needs surgery and I don't think it's a good idea to wait. She is already dehydrated and weak."

"And she needs a muzzle because she hurts so much." Marcy rubbed the doodle's ears, but Roxy didn't react.

She just looked at Marcy with sad eyes that nearly broke Violet's heart.

Marcy looked at her girl, pinched her eyes closed, sucked in a sob, then straightened her shoulders. When she opened her eyes, they were brimming with tears, but there was a resolution in them.

"I can't afford more than two thousand dollars." She pushed a tear away from her cheek. "I know how much these operations cost." Marcy's bottom lip quivered. "She's my best friend. I don't want to put her down, but I can't afford…"

Marcy sobbed, but she didn't drop her shoulders or look away from Violet. "If it is more than that, I need to talk about what we can do to end her suffering."

It was more, significantly more. But Roxy was well loved. Marcy was kicking her no-good boyfriend to the curb. Violet couldn't let her lose her best friend too.

"It's fifteen hundred. For all the medicine and surgery and everything." She saw Beck's head snap in her direction, but she didn't look at him.

"I can do that. I can do that. Oh. We will be eating peanut butter and jelly and mac and cheese for months. But it will be worth it." Macy kissed Roxy's head. "When?"

"Beck will get her prepped now. She will stay with us through tonight and maybe all of tomorrow. I know it is hard, but you should go home. Get some sleep."

"And hire a locksmith," Beck offered. "Seriously, if you kick Trevor out, hire one to make sure he can't get back in."

"No need." Marcy kissed Roxy one more time. "I can do that myself. My mother made sure I knew how. I'll stop at the hardware store as soon as they open."

"Good for her." Beck went the cabinet and grabbed the clippers they used to shave the fur where they'd put the IV port.

Yes, it was. The only recommendation Violet's mother ever gave her was to stay away from men. Advice she'd adhered to after Thomas's stunt. But that wasn't the right answer either.

Life was full of love and loss, joy and grief. The main thing you had to do was get out before you got your heart stomped on.

Her eyes found Beck. He wouldn't stomp on her heart. *Would he?*

"I'm going to get myself prepped." She headed for the door before she let her brain wander any further down that path. Beck had made it clear. He didn't plan to marry. Hell, he even had a rule about it.

And she wanted a life partner. Wanted the boring photo.

But not yet. She wasn't ready to give up the fun she was having with Beck.

There's still an expiration date.

That thought was going to get harder to ignore. She knew that, but that was future Violet's problem. She'd deal with the loss when it was time. For now she didn't want to let him go.

"Should we take an over under on the number of socks in Roxy's belly?" Vi stepped up to the operating table where Beck had prepped the large dog for her surgery.

"We both saw the X-ray. It's at least three and maybe as many as five." Beck never underestimated a big dog's ability to scarf down a whole host of things it shouldn't. "We'd be betting the same thing."

"True. We are on the same wavelength on that."

"Same wavelength." Beck chuckled. "My dad used to say that to my mom."

"Ah."

The soft sound sent a ripple of want through him. Same

wavelength. For a second it almost felt like his dad was over his shoulder cheering him on. He really would have loved Vi.

"First incision completed." Violet looked to him, her dark eyes catching his.

"All her vitals are stable."

"Right. Then now we get to the moment of truth." She made the next incision and let out a grunt. One sock, then another, and another and another. Four total. And a small ball. "That—" Violet held up the hacky sack ball "—started all of this."

"If Marcy wasn't going to break up with Trevor for the other reasons already, that would do it." Beck shook his head. "I swear the bar is so low for men sometimes."

"Nice to hear a man say that." Vi glared at the hacky sack ball one more time, then tossed it aside. "A little weird, but nice."

Beck kept his eyes on the monitors in front of him. He didn't think it was weird, but he'd heard more than one woman he dated mention that his views were a pleasant surprise.

People deserved partners who were present. Who saw what they needed and acted. It wasn't magic and the fact that a not-as-small-as-he'd-like subset of men felt that they were entitled to more even though they couldn't manage the minimum was frustrating as hell.

"You are pretty perfect, ya know." Vi was smiling behind her mask as she met his gaze.

Perfect. Heat bloomed on his skin, and his heart raced. Perfect.

Before he could work through the funnel of emotions bearing down on him, the monitor's alarms started going off.

"Oxygen is dropping," Beck called as he adjusted the oxygen flow for Roxy. "Heart rate decreasing. She's reacting to the anesthesia."

"Come on, Roxy," Vi muttered as she worked to keep the dog alive. "Your mommy needs you to snuggle, and beg for food. Actual food. Not socks."

Vi was panting as she finished the surgery as quickly as possible. Some dogs reacted to anesthesia. If they could close her up and wean her from the drugs, she might start responding.

"Closed, increase O2 and start to pull her off the anesthesia." Vi watched the numbers as Beck made the requested changes.

Roxy's heart rate started to come up but not as fast as he'd like to see.

Beck held his breath and looked at Vi. She was clearly thinking the same thing.

"Up the oxygen one more time."

He did as she instructed and let out a sigh as the dog finally started to respond.

"Yes. Yes." Violet leaned over and pressed a hug to him. "We did it."

"We did."

CHAPTER TWELVE

HE COULDN'T STOP tapping the wheel as he drove them to Mitch's studio. The date he'd planned for last week was finally happening. The surprise was the best he'd ever planned.

"You all right? You're nervously tapping that wheel." Vi laid a hand on his knee. "I'm going to love whatever you have planned."

"Yeah, you are." Beck grinned at her. She deserved so much. The woman looked after the needs of so many people. And animals. She wasn't taking any money for training the intermediate team. And Roxy had needed another surgery two days after they'd pulled the socks and ball from her intestine. Vi had covered that too.

Though Dr. Brown had given her a strong warning that the choice was kind, but it could bankrupt her if she wasn't careful.

Vi had told him that she'd accepted long ago that she'd rather just break even than turn away a loving owner. Plus she'd told Marcy it was a donor. It wasn't like everyone was going to assume it was her.

Bangor was a city with more than thirty thousand residents, but Beck suspected more than one pet owner knew it was Vi covering the expenses. If it leaked out, Dr. Brown might have a point.

"So sure of yourself." Violet leaned over and kissed his cheek. "That is quite the turn on, Beck."

"I'm not sure you really need any help getting turned on." Beck took one hand off the wheel and slowly traced his way up her thigh. They'd been inseparable since returning from Miami. She'd slept at his place nearly every day and gotten ready for their late shifts together.

It was homey. Maybe a little too homey, but he was doing his best to ignore the tiny voice in his head shouting that she was looking for a husband.

The studio was in the back of a rundown little area. Mitch, the stained-glass artist he'd found, had said it was so if there was ever a fire or explosion, unlikely but not impossible with the heat he was working with, it would limit the damage.

"Where are we?" Vi leaned forward.

"I know it doesn't look like much but trust me." He'd stopped out here a few weeks ago and initially wondered if he'd wandered into the wrong place. But the inside of the studio was brilliant.

"I trust you." She unbuckled her seat belt as soon as the car was stopped. "I kind of thought we might be hiking given the requirements for my feet here." She looked around. "But I don't see any trails."

"The reasons for the shoes will be clear in just a moment, I promise."

"Beck!" Mitch called as he stepped out of his studio. The aged hippy had long white hair pulled into low ponytail. He was wearing a heavy apron and his cheeks were rosy.

Stepping up to them, Mitch offered a hand to Beck, then turned to Violet. "And you must be the artist."

"Umm." Vi looked from Mitch to Beck, then shook her head. "I'm no artist."

"Sure you are. You're human. That means you're an artist." Mitch clapped and motioned for them to follow him.

"Trust me," Beck repeated. When he'd finally gotten Mitch to return his phone call, the retired art teacher had waxed poetically about art and creativity for nearly ten minutes before launching into the training program for stained glass.

He'd told Beck the reason was that anyone lacking the patience required for stained glass was going to hang up before the ten-minute mark. A unique strategy but if it worked for the man, who was he to judge?

"Oh my God." Violet put her hand over her mouth as she stepped into the art studio.

Stained glass hung in all the back windows—Mitch had called those his bad stock—not sellable. Beck had no idea what imperfections Mitch saw. All he could see was beauty.

"We are having a stained-glass lesson?" Violet looked at him, her eyes filled with tears.

"Vi. It's okay. We don't have to. Why are you crying?" This was supposed to make her happy. What had he done wrong?

"I don't know." She bit her lip and looked at the floor as she pushed the tears away. "I'm not sad. Just...overwhelmed. This is the absolute sweetest thing anyone has ever done for me."

"Yes. Yes. It is very sweet. I do not normally take students. So are we learning art today?" Mitch clapped his hands and Violet snapped to attention.

"Yes. We are learning art today." She did a little happy dance and moved over to where Mitch was standing.

Why the tears? All he'd wanted was to make her happy. And it had, but for a split second her tears were sad not happy. He was nearly sure of it.

"Oh. I get to pick a design. How fun." That was the bright happy Vi voice he was used to.

He looked at her and Mitch and his heart jumped.

He loved her.

Beck put a hand on his throat. How had that happened?

He wanted to mentally shake himself. It had happened because Vi was Vi. She was funny, kind, exciting, smart and gorgeous. She was the easiest person in the world to fall in love with.

Settling down with her would be easy. He could do that, right? Maybe it was years earlier than he'd anticipated ever marrying. But Vi, Vi was worth it.

"Are you coming?" She looked at him. "I'm making the giant key chain."

"First time for that one." Mitch laughed and gave Beck a thumbs-up.

When he'd gone over the premade designs they'd have for options tonight, Beck had instantly pulled the giant key chain. Mitch had tried to talk him out of it. He only got five presets—and according to Mitch he'd created that design one night when he'd smoked a little too much marijuana. He left it in the selection pile as a silly reminder to himself.

Beck had known the instant he'd seen it that Vi would pick it. Pick it, love it, hang it…

Where would she hang it? Her apartment didn't have many windows. His place. Well, his place had plenty of natural light.

"Beck?" She raised her hands again showing the key chain. "Come pick or I will pick for you and we don't need two key chains."

She giggled as she turned back toward Mitch.

We.

Such a simple little word. One she'd probably used without any thought behind it. But he…he wanted to be part of that we.

As long as he could keep from entering the boring life.

Surely he and Vi and could win against what his father said was an inevitability of a settled life.

The key chain she'd set in place wasn't very pretty. Even though she knew it would shine in the sun, the imperfections were easy to see. And Violet didn't care at all.

She'd made it. Her first piece of stained glass. This was the best present.

Violet swallowed the unexpected pain that raised. This was supposed to be a fun outing. It *was* a fun outing. But the second she'd figured out what he planned, her soul had screamed with joy before her heart felt like it was bursting.

She'd pulled herself together.

Then Mitch had chuckled when she'd chosen the key chain. Apparently, Beck had picked it specifically with her in mind. A throwaway line about collecting them on her travels—a line she barely remembered saying—had resulted in this beautiful monstrosity before her.

No one else had ever listened so freely to her. Ever internalized the things she said.

She looked over at him, bent over his design. Her heart swelled and her soul cried out that he was meant to be hers. She loved him. When it happened, how, why. None of it mattered. The truth was simple and terribly complicated. She loved Beck Forester.

That wasn't supposed to happen in a fling. Though technically his rule had been no marriage not no falling in love.

Not falling in love was an unstated rule. One she'd broken—splintered.

Beck wasn't interested in long-term. And she understood. He was twenty-six. Sure other twenty-six-year-olds were celebrating five- or six-year anniversaries and having their second or more children. But it was still young when you looked at it.

He wasn't ready for that life. Might never be ready. And that was okay.

Violet had no interest in children. At least not human ones. She enjoyed snuggling her friends' little ones. And enjoyed passing them back when they needed a diaper change or had spit up. Her mothering ways were all focused on fur babies.

That part of life wasn't for her...but she was ready for commitment. Ready to take the next steps with someone.

And the man I love isn't.

"What do you think?" Beck held up the mushroom with a rabbit hiding under it. His looked about like hers did.

Violet held hers up. "We did pretty awesome for one lesson."

"Maybe after we've been doing it for a year." Beck chuckled.

"Are we going to do this for a year?" It was like her words were hanging in the heated air. Spinning out of control as they raced toward him.

"I—" Her mind was devoid of all things. She looked for Mitch. Maybe there was some question she could ask about stained glass. Something, anything.

But the aged art instructor had taken himself out for a smoke break. Of course.

"Do you want us to do this for a year?" Beck raised an eyebrow, his dimples looking so damn lovely even in the heat of the workstations.

"What are you asking?" This couldn't be happening. It wasn't happening.

"We never set a deadline on the fling. Never said it had to end at a certain time. It could go on."

"For a year?" Hope pressed against her chest. She wasn't the same person she'd been when they scheduled this fake dating.

Wasn't the same person who'd gotten on the flight to Miami. No, that wasn't fair. It was the "Monster Mash" song. Winning the bet had awakened something in her. Reignited the spark she hadn't felt in so long.

"Or longer." Beck winked.

Tears pricked her eyes again. But this time it was joy racing through her.

"Or longer." Vi leaned across the bench and kissed him.

CHAPTER THIRTEEN

"I THINK MY face paint is scaring Larry the parrot. The bird keeps cursing at me anytime I pass his cage. And not his usual stuff either. Really foul innuendoes." Lacey glared back at the cage where the parrot was staying for the next four nights.

Dr. Brown didn't typically let patients board for nonemergency issues, but Larry had a habit of tricking anyone his owner, Mandy asked—or bribed—to look after the twenty-year-old African Grey.

His first owner, a creep Violet had—lucky for him—never met, had left the bird to its own devices and it had learned a lifetime of destructive habits. Mandy had dated Mr. No One Mentions His Name and taken Larry with her when they'd split less than four months later. The bird loved Mandy. He tolerated Dr. Brown.

The rest of the people in this world were things for him to squawk foul language at, scratch or bite.

"I don't think it is your Halloween makeup. And even if it is, that just means Larry is a bad judge of character. You are the cutest orange cat." It was truly impressive. Lacey had painted her face orange and then added the white lines you usually saw on orange tabby cats. The woman looked like a life-size orange cat.

Thankfully Lacey wasn't up to the mischief that orange kitties seemed incapable of not finding.

"I am pretty proud of this one." Lacey smiled. "But mostly I am proud that you showed up in costume tonight." She clapped as she pointed to the orange scrub top, red scrub bottoms that she'd rolled up to reveal knee high orange socks. "That Velma from Scooby Doo costume is perfect!"

It wasn't exactly a Velma costume, but given her role as an emergency vet, the full costume wasn't hugely practical.

"Thanks." She'd pulled it together after Beck had suggested they have a couple's costume. He had all the items for Fred and she had the items for Velma. It was a quick find but it was fun standing in the mirror at his place in the joint costume.

He was handing out candy until his shift started, and she was more than a little excited to see Lacey's reaction to his matching costume. They were dating; everyone knew and no one seemed surprised.

It was going well. And they were certainly staying busy. When they weren't training at the agility gym, Beck had something up his sleeve. In the week since they'd visited Mitch's stained-glass studio, they'd gone hiking—twice—and spent their free night on a ghost hunt. It was fun…and exhausting.

Beck always had an idea. A game plan. Something fun to do. She loved Bangor; it was a beautiful city. But it wasn't what one would call a hub of nightlife. Yet, Beck seemed to have an endless supply of ideas. He was talking about skydiving when the winter was over, and a weekend trip to Canada as soon as her passport was updated.

Like he is worried I'll get bored. Or he will.

That was a useless thought. They were dating. Having fun together and getting to know each other. He'd mentioned still being together in a year. A year was not a fling. A year was commitment.

"Fred's here!" Beck strode through the back entrance, in blue scrub pants, a white top, with an orange bandanna around his neck.

"You guys match." Lacey did a little happy dance. "Oh. That is so cute."

"And you make the perfect orange cat, except you are far too brilliant." Beck winked.

Lacey stuck her tongue out at him. "Just because all of them seem to share the same brain cell is no reason to pick on them." She folded her arms but failed to keep a straight face. "At least they are cute."

"They do have that going for them." Beck nodded and headed to the sink to wash up.

A squawk followed by a stream of unpleasant language echoed around them.

"Good evening to you too, Larry."

A bell rang and Lacey darted to the reception desk.

Violet wandered over to Beck, leaned against the sink beside him and kissed his cheek. "You were right, even with the scrubs, everyone knows we are Fred and Velma."

He brushed his lips past hers, the touch barely there. "It is the spirit of the night, not the costume. Plus anyone who isn't frantic when they come in here tonight will pay us no attention when they see Lacey. Seriously, she is a master with the makeup."

It wasn't a competition, but he was right. If it was, their receptionist was taking all the prizes.

"How many kids did you pass out candy to?" She'd been shocked by how much candy he'd procured for the evening, particularly since her shift started as trick or treat began, and his started before it was over.

"About thirty. Not bad for an hour."

"I used to love trick or treating. My friends and I would take pillowcases and do our best to fill them with all sorts of treats. I bet I walked two to three miles every Halloween. We did it well into our teen years when we were the biggest kids out there." Those were some of her best childhood memories.

Her parents had never cared to come with her. They bought a costume at a local box store or told her to find something in her closet. She'd gone as a black cat at least four years in a row.

"I never got to go." Beck cleared his throat as he moved away from the counter.

"What?" He'd spent nearly twenty minutes in the grocery store trying to pick out candy. He'd gone back and forth between a few bags, before she'd just dumped both in their cart and told him they could always put extra out at the clinic. It would disappear faster than one could say abracadabra.

"Halloween is one of the most dangerous nights of the year for a kid." Beck shrugged.

That was probably true. It was nighttime and kids were running around, many like her, unsupervised. But the stat had to be skewed too. Because it was the one night where a large majority of children were all doing the same thing.

"On average children are twice as likely to be hit by a car and killed on Halloween than any other day of the year. Many of the costumes are cheap and fire hazards or contain dangerous levels of toxins. And of course jack-o'-lanterns start an average of nine hundred house fires a year."

Violet blinked, not quite sure what to do with that sobering information.

"I heard that every year. Every year, when I asked for a costume or begged to go trick or treating. I told them once that millions of children trick or treat each year and while the loss of any life was tragic the odds were in my favor." Beck frowned as he looked down at his shoes, clearly not sure what to do with himself.

"What did they say when you pointed it out?" She wished he'd said this when they were buying candy. Wished he'd pointed it out when talking about costumes. Wished they were anywhere other than work with a patient checking in. He needed to be held. Needed to get out whatever anger or frustration was brewing under that statement.

"They were excellent statisticians. They worked out the odds and decided it was too much. They loved me so much they weren't willing to risk it."

"Beck."

"They loved me. Treasured me. I know that. I know I sound bratty for even caring about trick or treating."

"You don't." He'd been loved and smothered. Two things could be true at once.

"I need to triage the patient. Hopefully, it's nothing serious."

He left before she could say anything else. But what else was there to say?

A lot. Just not here at the clinic.

"I looked away for a split second and she grabbed the candy from my hand. I got it back but she ate some chocolate and…" Belle Sanchez was running her hands over the black Lab mix that she'd brought home from the shelter less than four days ago. "Lucky, I am so sorry."

Belle hiccupped as the dog wagged its tail.

"Take a deep breath for me." Beck wasn't overly worried about Lucky. Chocolate toxicity was a threat, but Lucky weighed over forty pounds. Serious toxicity usually set in after they ate more than half an ounce per pound of their body weight. In Lucky's situation that meant twenty ounces, which was several full-size candy bars. It was always possible there were underlying conditions or that the dog might have an unknown allergy but part of a snack size candy bar was not overly a concern as long as Lucky continued to the act like she was perfectly fine.

Lucky licked Belle's face and put her paws on her shoulders as her owner continued to cry.

"Breathe for me, Belle. Lucky is fine."

"Chocolate toxicity can take up to twelve hours to show up." Belle bit her lip as she looked at her watch. "It might just be too soon."

The internet provided a lot of good information. Information he was glad the general population had access too. However, particularly for people with anxious personalities, it could come with a host of worries.

He pressed the button on the side of the cabinet that would alert Vi that he needed her in the room right now. Unfortunately, there wasn't a way to alert her that the issue was the pet parent not the pet.

Belle was spinning, worrying that she'd done something wrong. And he suspected that she'd read every horrid thing that might happen with chocolate toxicity.

His mom had googled the stats for every activity before he was allowed to participate. Football—concussion risk. That one was fair. And as more data was coming, he even understood her worries. Swimming—drowning risk. Except you were infinitely more likely to drown if you were scared of the water or didn't know how to swim.

Trick or treating…

That one still upset him. He'd missed out on such a common experience of childhood. And the truth was the activity was quite safe if the parents or guardians paid attention.

"Lucky had very little chocolate. You did a good job." Beck kept his voice soft, but firm. She'd done exactly right. Gotten the chocolate from the dog and started monitoring.

"What seems to be the problem?" Vi walked in, so cute in her scrub Velma outfit.

He'd never done a couple's costume. Never wanted to. But when she'd mentioned finding something for the evening it had popped out. It would have been better for it to pop out at least a day before their Halloween shift, but they'd made it work.

"Lucky gobbled chocolate." Belle sobbed as she buried her head in the dog's coat.

"Not exactly accurate." Beck handed Vi the notes he'd written up. "Lucky had a part, a small part, of a snack size candy bar. Belle acted fast and got it away from him, but she is worried about chocolate toxicity."

"The internet—"

"Is full of scary things about dogs and chocolate." Vi interrupted, stepping up to the exam table. "I am not saying it isn't real—it very much is. But it takes a lot of chocolate for a dog this size to succumb to it. Even if you had a teacup Chihuahua, we wouldn't panic unless it ate the whole bite sized piece and was showing symptoms."

"But it can take time." Belle was repeating exactly what she'd told him.

Maybe Vi could relieve her worries.

Though once his mom had started an anxiety spiral it sometimes took days for her to come out of it.

"It can. But Lucky is acting perfectly fine." Violet held up a hand. "Let me explain what you should be looking for…"

Vi began to outline the symptoms of chocolate toxicity, asking Belle if Lucky was exhibiting any of them. With each negative response, Belle seemed to take a deeper breath.

"So you think she will be okay?"

"I do." Violet nodded. "She is very lucky to have you. It was a good name choice."

"The shelter chose it. I didn't think it was kind to change a name she was already responding too." Belle ran her hand down Lucky's back.

Dogs didn't really care what their humans called them, provided they were rewarded with love, food, play and the occasional treat. He'd let more than one pet parent know they didn't have to keep the name a shelter or previous owner gave their pet. But they absolutely could too. There was not a right or wrong answer with a name.

"I always wanted a dog, but my parents were very against animals in the house." Belle kissed the top of Lucky's head. "I had a dog, Misty, that my parents made me leave in the backyard."

Beck saw Violet shudder. Dogs could and should enjoy being outside. But, unless they were guardian livestock animals, then they needed to have a place in the home too.

"One night when it was snowing so hard, I snuck Misty into my room. It was so cold…and when my mom found her the next morning, well, Misty went to live with someone else then."

"I am so sorry, Mandy." There was nothing else he could say. He wasn't surprised. A cold truth of working in veterinary medicine was learning that many people should never have pets.

But Mandy was not one of those people.

"I saw Lucky on the shelter site and knew she was mine. I know that sounds weird but the picture…she was looking into the camera and I just had to go get her, and then I have her less than a week and I feed her chocolate."

"No." Vi shook her head. "You did *not* feed her chocolate. She took it from your hand and you immediately reacted and then got her seen by a vet. You did everything right, Mandy."

Mandy looked from Vi to Beck. He nodded. "She is right. That is why she has fancy degree hanging behind the receptionist's desk."

"You really think she's going to be all right?" Mandy looked at Lucky like she was trying to peer into her gut to find the exact amount of the offending candy.

"I do, but we'll give you a list of things to look for over the next twelve hours. If you see her reacting in any of the ways outlined, then you bring her back and we'll go from there. But you were a good dog mom today." Vi stepped up to Mandy. "Do you want a hug?"

Mandy stepped into Vi's arms. Not enjoying being left out of the affection, Lucky let out a bark and tilted her head as she surveyed the women.

"Thank you. I was just so worried." Mandy wiped a tear from her cheek as she stepped back.

"One thing that might help is getting her into training. There are basic dog training classes offered at the Happy Feet Gym or you can learn a lot through online videos." Beck had used online videos for Toaster's initial trainings. "The biggest things you want her to have without fail is 'leave it,' so she doesn't take food or other items that are bad for her, 'stay,' so she doesn't move from the place you need her and 'drop it'… in case she doesn't follow number one as well as possible."

"But—" Vi pointed a finger "—we don't go down rabbit hole videos of terrible things that might happen to our puppy. We live in the present. Not worrying about a future that is out of our control. Right?"

"Right." Mandy nodded, but he could see that she wasn't 100 percent behind following that advice. The woman was going to google and he doubted this was the first time they'd see Lucky in the ER for a minor thing.

"Beck will get you all set up with the signs and symptoms and if you have concerns, call the clinic." Violet offered her one more smile before stepping out of the room.

He gave Mandy the information packets on training, what to look for with chocolate toxicity. Lucky wagged her tail, happy to be headed home as they walked through the door.

As he stepped into the back room, Vi looked up. "Do you think I calmed her down?"

"Yes. For how long? I don't know." Beck blew out a breath and looked at the closed door. His mother had heard from countless doctors that Beck was fine. That playing sports was good for him. That independence was something to cultivate.

But she'd been too scared to risk losing the son she'd waited so long for.

Now he did it all.

"I can fix so many things, even mild to severe chocolate toxicity. But I can't fix a worried pet parent who is just trying to do their best."

There wasn't anyone else back here, and there were no patients actively waiting on them. Beck pulled her to him, kissing the top of her head.

"We do the best we can, Vi."

She looked up at him, her dark gaze smoky in the matching costume to his.

"Think there will be any candy left to dig into when we get home?"

Home. She'd referred to his place as home. He smiled, enjoying the simple phrase. "I think so. Someone made me buy far too much candy."

CHAPTER FOURTEEN

BEAR FLOPPED ON the floor next to Toaster, who opened an eye but didn't bother to get up. As soon as Beck mentioned getting her run in, the border collie mix would focus on nothing else, but at least for the moment she was willing to just relax.

"I feel the exact same way, guys." Violet took off her shoes and hung her coat up on the rack Beck had by the door. All she wanted tonight was to order in and stream some mindless television show.

It wasn't that the Halloween shift had been bad. It had simply been a steady stream. All of the animals they'd seen tonight were either already going home with their owners or headed there after short stays at the clinic. That was a good thing, but it didn't mean her battery wasn't drained after moving from one crisis to another.

"So, I was thinking that tomorrow we might go to the Rock Shop. They are having a discussion on natural history." Beck bounced into the room, holding two mugs of decaf coffee. "Or we could rent some bikes and go—"

"Or we could stay home and rest." Violet interrupted, as she took her cup of coffee from his hands. "Thank you."

She held the mug up to her lips enjoying the smell and the warmth in her hands. She had a strict rule about caffeine after her night shifts. If there was any hope of her maintaining some kind of regular sleep schedule, she couldn't have it just after her shift.

No matter how much she craved it.

"We could take a day off." Beck leaned forward his lips brushing hers.

The touch sent fire through her, but his words froze her heart. "Beck, we do not have to always be doing something." She had a better understanding of why he felt the need to try new things after what he said about his mother not letting him try anything.

Including trick or treating. Outside of Christmas that was the best holiday as a kid. The one night a year you were allowed to take candy from strangers.

Being told that was too risky would leave a mark on anyone. Even make them thrilled to jump on a plane and go to a wedding with a colleague as a fake date.

Spontaneity and an openness to try new things were good traits. But just like his parents, it was possible to swing too far the other way.

"Sure, we don't have to, but we don't want to become boring immediately." He took a sip of his coffee and snapped his fingers.

Toaster popped to attention and moved toward the back door.

"While I take her for her agility run, why don't you find something for us to binge on our boring night." Beck moved to follow Toaster.

"Watching television does not have to be boring," Violet called out as she heard the back door open.

Boring. That was his focus. Or rather the thing he was trying to avoid at all costs in life.

She looked at the television, picked up the remote then set

it down. Toaster and Beck would be on his makeshift course outside burning off her energy for at least thirty minutes.

She wanted another look at the boring picture—as he called it. Maybe she'd missed something when she'd looked at it the first time. Maybe there was a clearer meaning to why it bothered him so much.

An answer to why he couldn't just relax in their relationship.

Beck took one more breath of fresh air as Toaster rounded the corner of the A-Frame. His girl had run for a solid thirty minutes. And he'd used every one of those seconds to beat himself up.

They'd had a long night. Two dogs had gotten loose and tangled in chicken coop wire a neighbor had left out, resulting in deep cuts to one's hind legs and the other's abdomen. A dog had come in after eating a bag of candy—and unlike Lucky they'd had to induce vomiting and were keeping the poor guy overnight to watch for chocolate toxicity. And just before their shift ended, a cat with smoke inhalation from a barn fire had been rushed in by a farmer, whose night had gone from fun Halloween games to nightmare.

The animals were all going to recover. Not a thing he got to say about every shift. But the hug they'd shared after talking to Mandy was the last moment of free time they'd gotten.

And he was complaining about spending the rest of the day sleeping, watching mindless television and cuddling with the woman he loved.

Get a grip, Beck!

Toaster panted at his side, waiting for the command to run the backyard course again or to go in.

"Let's go see what Vi picked out." Beck snapped two fingers and Toaster turned and walked to the back door.

She stopped at the water bowl while he continued to the living room. The screen was dark. The couch empty.

Bear was lying on his bed.

"Where is your mom, Bear?"

The pittie opened his eyes, let out a yawn but gave no further indication to where Vi might be hiding.

Stepping into the hallway he froze. Light poured out from under the crack in his parents' study. "Vi?"

"I'm in the study," she called back.

He knew that. But had hoped she might pop out and explain why she was spending any time in there when she could be curled on the couch with a pittie. Instead, he was going to have to go into the one room in the house he disliked.

Once upon a time he'd loved the study. Loved sitting at his parents' feet while they worked and talked. They'd chatted continuously. About important things, nothings, and everything in between.

When his father died, the room had quieted and when his mother had to move into a full-time care facility, it had silenced forever.

"What are you doing in here?"

"Looking at photos." Vi held up a box with prints from his parents' years together.

"Some of these are great. You should put them in frames. Or maybe we could take a scrapbooking class. This one should be in a frame!" She smiled up at him as she held up a photo of his mom and dad in the kitchen. His mom holding a beer while his father cooked.

The irony of the photo taken in the late eighties with the

gender roles swapped was not lost on him. But it certainly wasn't frame worthy. It was just a picture of how they'd been.

His father had joked that he'd had to learn to cook because his mother had no ability to do it and no willingness to learn. She'd always laughed at that and told his dad there was no reason to learn when she'd married a master.

"Seriously, Beck." Violet reached for another picture, but he picked up the box before she could.

"These are nothing. They are just day-to-day pics. Nothing exciting."

"That isn't true." Vi crossed her arms, shaking her head. "These are exciting in their own way."

"Exciting." Beck put the box on his dad's desk and grabbed her hand. "I'll show you exciting." He pulled her to the hallway where he'd framed an image of his father on top of a mountain.

"And this one—" he pointed to a hiking picture "—this is exciting."

Turning, he pointed to another image, this one of his father on an archaeological dig. One of the few archaeological digs he'd taken part in after he'd married Beck's mother. Those trips dwindled away, and the rest was boring history. "This was one of Dad's last digs. Do you know how old he was?"

Vi squeezed his hand. "Beck."

"Seriously, Vi. How old do you think he is here."

"Thirty-five?"

"Nope. Twenty-nine. Twenty-nine years old. Do you know how many digs he could have gone on? How many trips he just didn't even try for? And why?"

"Because he loved your mother." Her face fell as she said the words.

"No." That was the rub of it. He didn't think their love had anything to do with it. It was the marriage certificate. The piece of paper that made them one in the eyes of the government that had changed them. "It was marriage."

Vi opened her mouth, then shut it. She crossed her arms, rocking back, her eyes glued to the floor in front of her.

Away from me.

The space between them was less than three feet but crossing it seemed impossible.

"My parents argued every single day. They screamed at each other. Threw things. Blamed me for their lot in life."

"Vi—"

Her gaze rooted to the floor. "I don't have a single photo of them happy. My dad burned the wedding photos after an argument. My mother ripped up the pictures of their early years after another."

She wiped at a tear on her cheek. "Maybe that's why I think a cooking photo or a garden party where two people seem content with each other in a crowd of people is so exciting."

Beck swallowed, hoping it might free the words caught in his throat. This was a crossroad. A junction. A point that shifted everything.

"Sorry I barged in here. I was—" Vi finally looked up, but instead of looking at him, she let her gaze wander around the room. "I don't actually know what I was thinking."

"Movie time?" The suggestion sounded a little hollow on his lips, but Vi smiled. Not a full smile but a smile.

"Sure. We should order some food too. I'm hungry and neither of us are master cooks." She hit his hip with hers, but the motion he'd come to enjoy so much over the last couple of weeks didn't have the oomph behind it.

"Did you cut your hair?" Nikki tilted her head as she looked at Violet. The owner of one of the local hair shops was always fishing for her to come in and let her play with her color. Nikki was currently sporting a bright red bob with junky blond highlights. It wasn't Violet's cup of tea, but if it made her happy then that was what mattered.

"Nope. I have an appointment with my regular gal in a week or so just to trim the dead ends." Violet blew a loose strand of hair out of her eyes. She was going to pull it back into a bun shortly. She seemed to start some shifts with the idea that today was the day she just left it down. And halfway through, or sometimes minutes into her shift, she just lost it and yanked it into a ponytail or messy bun.

"Well, I think you'd rock a blond, or maybe even some purple. Mix it up."

Violet made a noncommittal sound, hoping Nikki would launch into the pet-related reason she was here.

"Something about you is different." Nikki looked at Beck, then pointed at her. "Don't you think something is different?"

Beck grinned. He knew exactly what was different with her. Knew that she was waking up satisfied in his bed. Coming out of the shell she'd wrapped herself in when Thomas left her at the altar. It was a rebirth, and she was enjoying every minute.

Well, nearly every minute.

Their argument two nights ago was still stuck in her head. Argument, fight, misunderstanding…all of those words seemed too much of a descriptor.

And yet somehow not enough.

She'd give almost anything to have a love like his parents. They glowed in the photos. People she'd never get to meet, who'd created the sweetest man she'd ever known.

And he didn't want what they'd had. Scorned it even.

"You are sure you didn't cut your hair?" Nikki looked at her. "You just have that something fresh vibe going on."

"I think I would know if I cut it," Violet laughed. "But we aren't here to talk about my hair." She took in the large male tabby very unhappy to be in the carrier Nikki had him in.

Nikki looked at her giant orange cat and smiled. "He'll calm down as soon as I get him out." She unzipped the carrier top, lifted the giant up and sat him on her shoulder.

"We just sent an angry parrot home, and I would have loved to snap a picture of Larry on a shoulder and then have Frank on yours." Beck let out a chuckle as the orange tabby ran his head along Nikki's.

"Yeah, my husband started this when he was a kitten. It was cute when he weighed five pounds. Even when he weighed ten…but at seventeen it can be a bit much." Nikki ran a hand along Frank's back, and the cat let out a satisfied rumble.

"You told Beck he was here because of a string missing from your sewing basket."

"I have looked all over for it." Nikki playfully glared at Frank. "And given his history…"

Frank had consumed about six inches of fishing line two years ago. It had wrapped around the back of his tongue as it moved through his intestines requiring emergency surgery and several nights at the clinic.

Cats were typically better than dogs at not eating inedible items, except for string. There was something about the movement of it that made their predator instincts flare.

Violet wasn't exactly sure what caused it, but she'd removed as much string from cats in her career as she had socks from dogs.

"But you aren't sure he ate it." Beck added as he pulled up

the X-ray. "There is nothing there, but that doesn't necessarily mean anything."

She looked at the X-ray. If Frank had eaten the string a few hours ago, there was little the images could provide and it was too soon to see a blockage.

"I think our best bet is to administer a purgative." That would clear Frank's stomach and hopefully pull up any string he'd eaten.

Beck left to get the medication.

"While Beck is gone, let's just go over what will happen."

"You're going to make him throw up." Nikki shrugged and Frank let out a meow at the shift in his perch. "This is not his first rodeo on these. Honestly that is the cheapest option, though he is going to be pissed."

Violet smiled as she ran a hand over Frank's ears. The massive boy rumbled and pushed his head against her hand. "You aren't going to like me for much longer. I should get the attention while I can. Or maybe I should make Beck do it."

"Maybe you should." Nikki giggled as she pulled Frank off her shoulders and cradled the cat in her arms. If Frank minded the change in his position, he did not show it.

"So, while we wait, let's get back to you. It's not your hair and you aren't wearing makeup." Nikki squinted at her, then her mouth widened. "You're dating someone."

"I am." Heat poured over her cheeks. Violet knew Nikki from the clinic, and while Bangor was one of the largest cities in Maine, it still felt like a small town sometimes. Maybe if she knew something was different she'd move on.

"I'm very happy." Violet plastered a smile on, hoping Beck would be back with the medication shortly. She liked Nikki as a client. The woman loved Frank, which was what was most important. But she didn't know her well enough to talk about her relationship.

"Ooh." Nikki clapped. "Maybe we will be seeing you in a white dress soon?"

"Maybe," Violet offered as the door opened. She'd learned when she first arrived in Bangor that if she didn't want to carry on the conversation, *maybe* was the best way to curtail the conversation.

A *yes* or *no* seemed to bring on advice. Or questions to try to get her to dive in deeper. A *maybe* was wishy-washy enough that the person she was talking to could reasonably assume she agreed with them, even if she didn't.

Beck handed her the medicine, and there was the ghost of question in his eyes.

"Was there a problem finding this?" She looked at the box, checking the expiration date and the dosage. Beck would have done that too, but it was protocol for the techs and the vets to each check.

He looked at Frank and then Nikki, but not at her. "No. I just had to make sure we had enough for him. He is a bit of a big guy." Beck pulled on the long heavy gloves and took a deep breath. Frank was a sweet boy, but no cat liked having a syringe shoved down his throat.

Before Frank could make sense of what happened, Beck had him pinned. The yowls started immediately.

"I did warn you that you were going to be mad at me." Violet quickly slid the medicine behind his tongue, pushed it out then closed his mouth, forcing Frank to swallow.

If the feline could speak, the curses might even make Larry the parrot blush.

Beck let go as soon as the medicine was in and Frank took off. He was under the bench, glaring at all of them.

"So now we wait thirty minutes and see if it works, right?" Nikki crossed her arms as she looked at the angry orange creature she'd brought in.

"Like you said, it's not his first rodeo. So you know the routine. If he starts to do anything, I want you to push this button and I will come to make sure it goes as smoothly as possible." Cats were notoriously difficult patients. They rarely showed symptoms until it was almost too late and unlike dogs, induced vomiting did not have a high success rate.

"I will. And if you ever want to talk about the hunk you are planning to meet at the altar, you let me know. And keep me in mind when you need wedding updos. I give group rates." Nikki sat on the bench, pulling her legs up quickly as Frank swatted at them.

They were certainly personae non gratae with the usually friendly feline.

"Okay." Violet waved as she headed back through the door. As Beck closed it, she held up her hands. "I haven't been planning or scheming a way to get you to the altar. I know we aren't going there. I just didn't want to discuss it and I said maybe and Nikki assumed and—" Her words ran out as he shrugged.

"It's not a big deal, Vi." He kissed her cheek. "You want to get married someday and I don't plan to. But we are having fun now." He winked, then moved off to the patient in the next room.

Violet buried her hands in her scrubs pocket, her fingernails cutting into her palms as she balled her hands. She was trying to explain and he'd shrugged it off. But not because he was worried she was trying to force the issue he'd said was a nonstarter.

He'd indicated he saw them together. Indicated they had a future.

She wasn't overly concerned about a wedding license. Marriage wasn't the only way to commit to someone. But he saw an end date for them. A final point. Not today or even this year, but he expected their chapter to close.

Pinching her eyes closed she willed the tears away. There was a time for them. And there were going to be a lot of them—soon. But not here.

Not yet.

CHAPTER FIFTEEN

BECK RACED ALONG the weave poles, cringing as Toaster missed the third one again. How was that possible? Weave poles were her favorite obstacle.

The agility competition was this weekend. He knew Violet was trying to pretend that she didn't care about whether their team placed. Knew she was actively avoiding any thoughts of running into Thomas.

Which was 100 percent going to happen since the man seemed hell-bent on seeking them out at his stepbrother's wedding. He could only imagine what it was going to be like when they were on his "turf" so to speak.

"Beck." Vi's voice was firm as it hit him from the other side of the gym.

So she'd seen the mess up—again.

He was hoping she was focused on Tim or Lacey. She probably had been, but the woman seemed to pick up everything in the agility gym. It was like her radar pinged every time perfection slipped away.

"I know. I know." He held up his hand. "Toaster faulted on the weave poles. We'll run it again." He gave the command for Toaster to follow him back to the start of the obstacle.

She let out a soft whine but followed the command.

Before he could get her started, Vi raced over. "Stop."

"What?" He crossed his arms, then immediately uncrossed them. "I mean what?"

He was touchy. Had been touchy since Nikki mentioned doing Vi's hair for her wedding.

No, it was Vi's explanation after. Her insistence that she didn't plan on marrying him. Nikki loved to play the matchmaker. Loved to do wedding hair and makeup. It was her salon's specialty, and she was always stumping for business. He hadn't thought that much of it—until Vi jumped to explain.

She wasn't planning on meeting him at the altar. It was what he'd asked for. What he wanted.

He had no reason to be bothered. But he couldn't seem to shake off the anxious thoughts.

She was pulling away. It wasn't much. A few less touches. An extra night stayed at her place.

With each day it was like they were slipping further away from each other. But neither was willing to acknowledge it. Maybe they were scared to.

Violet tilted her head, looking from him to Toaster. Then she sat on the ground and motioned for Toaster to come sit in her lap. It was one of Bear's favorite games. Despite the pittie's sixty-pound weight, Bear truly believed he was a lapdog.

Now Toaster felt the same was true for her.

"You are doing great, girl." Violet rubbed her face in Toaster's hair. Beck's dog wagged her tail so hard her whole body was moving.

"Not sure that is quite true. We've faulted each time on the run through the weave poles tonight." Beck crossed his arms as he stared at the obstacle. Usually it was a no-brainer for Toaster. Was it just that they hadn't practiced this one much that she was faltering?

Vi kissed Toaster's nose, then looked up at him. "It's not Toaster that's faulting, it's you."

Beck blinked, not sure what to say to that. "I'm running the course the same way I always do, Vi. Right down the center, snapping my fingers for her and calling out commands. We do this every night either here or in the backyard. Literally." There was nothing different now than there had been yesterday.

"You're stressed. And she is picking up on that." Violet swallowed and looked away. "If you want to talk about what is bugging you, we can do that."

"Not here we can't."

Vi nodded, and he saw her bite her lip. "So it is us." She kissed Toaster on the head one more time, then pushed herself up off the ground.

"Vi—" He hadn't meant to hurt her. That was never his goal. He loved her. Loved her so much.

But Thomas had been right. She wanted a husband. Deserved a husband. A quiet steady love. And he was holding her back.

So let her go.

The words blasted through his brain, but his heart refused to recognize them. How could you love someone and know you weren't there forever?

She could be.

His heart had refused to listen to his brain since day one with Vi.

"Violet. I have a question about helping Tuna with her banks. She is pushing off the center and dangerously close to the fault line."

She looked over to Lisa and Tuna, putting on her trainer

face. "We'll talk after practice." Vi looked at him, her smile breaking just a little before she jogged off to help Lisa.

"It's late and we have a long day tomorrow. What if we just put off the conversation until we wake up?"

Beck's offer was too good to pass up. Even though Vi knew they should hash it out now.

Coward.

She'd opened a chasm last week when she'd looked through his parents' things. And it had widened after Nikki's wedding jokes.

They were both walking on eggshells around the other. Both knowing what might be coming and neither willing to pull at the thread that was growing impossible to ignore.

"You hungry?"

"No." Violet dropped her bags by his front door. Her stomach was rolling too much to think of putting much sustenance in it. "You?"

"Not for food." Beck raised his eyebrows in the silly manner he had. It was a running joke they had. One they hadn't used since she'd gone through his parents' stuff. So many of their little fun things had ended after that.

Because it was the end of our fling.

That was the moment. The true moment this became a relationship. One doomed to fail.

Fiona had told her once when they were in college and she was dating some frat guy that she swore was fun but not forever that you either dated to marry or to break up.

"Beck." She pulled him close—clinging to him as she traced kisses down his neck. This wasn't what they should be doing, but Vi didn't care.

She needed another night with him. One more time with the man she loved. She could say goodbye tomorrow.

His arm wrapped around her waist, arching her toward him. "Vi."

Her name, whispered on his lips undid her.

"Take me to bed, Beck. Now."

Tomorrow. Tomorrow they'd talk. Tomorrow she'd figure out what the next steps were. Tomorrow she'd face heartbreak head-on.

But tonight was hers and Beck's. All theirs.

Beck rolled over and wasn't surprised to find the bed empty. Pulling a hand over his face, he stared at the ceiling. They'd spent the night cocooned in each other.

Each touch weighted with a meaning he didn't want to look at too closely in the morning light. They had today off. He'd planned to see if she wanted to go hiking again, or maybe to the market to see the Christmas decorations. The market had put up the trees and snowmen as soon as the trick-or-treaters had headed to bed.

Thanksgiving might be in between Halloween and Christmas, but no one was paying that holiday any attention.

Now though.

He heard Bear bark and a little worry slipped from him. Part of Beck had worried that she might disappear on him. Last night was the most intense night of his life, other than the first night he'd loved her.

They were together. Each anticipating the other's needs, the other's wants. But the last time. The last time they'd gone slow. Taking their time, memorizing everything about the other.

Saying goodbye with their bodies before they said it out loud.

She wanted marriage. She deserved marriage. She deserved someone who knew they wanted that life.

He got out of bed and looked around his room. Her stuff was gone. Beck slid his hand across the bedside table where her book and reading lamp had been sitting last night. Her clothes were no longer on the oversize chair in the corner.

He stood, knowing what he'd find in the bathroom and needing to see it anyway. Her makeup, toothbrush and hairbrush were no longer scattered on the extra sink. It was like she'd packed up all the pieces she'd left.

She was going to be the first to leave this time.

There were two options. Take his time getting ready, prolong what they'd already prolonged last night. Or rush through it and embrace the heartbreak waiting for him in the kitchen or living room. Neither option appealed to him, but hurrying ended the suspense fastest.

The aroma of coffee filled the hall on his way to the kitchen, and his mouth watered as he heard the bacon sizzling. If her things weren't gone from his room, he might assume this was just another day for them.

"Good morning, Violet." The words were thick as he took her in.

Her dark hair in a low ponytail; black leggings with a green sweater pulled over top. She had on long gray socks that if she put on boots could roll over the top. Vi looked ready to go the Christmas market.

But there was a look in her eyes. A hint of the conversation they'd put off last night.

Pulling the bacon from the skillet, she put it on a plate, then moved to the table and sat down while he fixed his coffee.

"Thanks for breakfast." Beck grabbed a slice of toast from a plate she must have set out before the bacon and took a bite.

He didn't expect a fight, but getting a meal and sitting down wasn't what he'd prepped for either.

"What was the issue last night?" Vi sipped her coffee, her dark gaze holding his. No accusation, just a question.

"You want to get married." He rolled his thumb on the edge of the table. "I don't."

"Have I said I want to get married?" Vi tilted her head, tapping her fingers against her plate.

"Not directly."

"So no." Vi took a deep breath. "Why do you think I want to meet anyone at the altar so badly? My one failed trip was a fairly large disaster."

"Thomas—"

Vi scooted back in her chair at the mention of her ex, crossing her arms. "Our relationship has nothing to do with Thomas."

"It does, actually. It has everything to do with him. He is the reason you were so shut up here in Bangor for years. He is the reason you didn't want to go alone to Miami. He is the reason you invited me. He is the reason…"

"Stop." Vi shook her head. "You being terrified of commitment has nothing to do with my ex. Yes, he was a catalyst but—"

"I saw you at Fiona's wedding, Vi." He wasn't afraid of commitment. One day, he'd probably settle down. Be the boring husband. He just wasn't ready to hang up the fun quite yet. "I watched you participate in the bouquet dance. I saw how disappointed you were when the bouquet went to someone else. Yes, you covered it quickly but it was there." He'd seen it. Real disappointment.

"I was disappointed." Vi shrugged. "I like to win and that was a fun bouquet. Fiona made it out of recycled brochures if you remember. Not exactly the usual kind of thing you get during a bouquet toss."

Beck blinked. Had he read that situation wrong? Built that moment into something more? "You want a relationship."

Vi nodded. "I thought that was what we had, but—"

She blew out a breath and looked out the window. He followed her gaze. His stained glass still hung there. Hers was gone. Another piece of herself she'd removed from his place while he slept.

"But you are right. We want different things. I want someone committed to me. Someone who sees a future with me. Someone who wants a quiet, steady love that is comfortable in the boring parts of life."

"So marriage."

"You are the only one using that term. I don't care about a ring or a piece of paper." Vi stood up, put both hands on her stomach. "I want someone who sees a future with me. Not someone who is terrified that by loving me, they will lose themselves. Your parents found themselves in love."

He opened his mouth, but she held up a hand.

"You are diminishing them by calling it boring. It was right for them." She grabbed her plate and mug and walked over to the sink.

"I think you've been looking for a reason I might leave since we decided to date. I mean all of your stuff is already packed up. Worried that I might try to keep something like Thomas did? You don't even know that I care about you enough to make sure you have everything you wanted."

Violet looked to the window where her stained-glass key chain had hung when they went to bed this morning. "I think we're agreed that we aren't a good match. We still have to work together and we are going to Boston soon. We are adults, this was a fling, so…"

She looked at him and he had no words.

Say something!

No. This is for the best.

Tell her you love her.

We want different things right now.

Do something.

His heart and his brain warred with each other as she pushed away from the counter, but he couldn't manage to work anything out.

He let her leave. Didn't run after her when the front door shut. This was the right thing.

So why did it feel like his soul left with her?

CHAPTER SIXTEEN

THREE DAYS. It had been three days since he'd let Vi walk out of this home. Toaster nuzzled his hand, and he rubbed the top of her head.

"I miss her too. Not that I haven't seen her every day." They'd worked two shifts together and done the final touches on the agility team yesterday. They'd professionally ignored each other.

That was the best description for the coolness between them. It wasn't just the light touches and stolen kisses in slow moments that he missed. It was the silly banter, the quick platonic hugs after tough cases. The simple conversations.

Even Lacey had mentioned that the temperature seemed to drop ten degrees every time they were in the room together. But what else was he supposed to do?

In two days the team would leave for Boston. Except instead of riding with him and Toaster down to the facility, Vi was carpooling with Nancy. The gym owner had Oliver in a few single competitions and had gladly offered Vi a ride so she didn't have to drive by herself.

He suspected Nancy would spend the entire time chatting about training manuals, techniques and all things agility. Given that they were rooming together, Nancy was going to have a lot of time to pick Vi's brain. Clearly, Vi would do *anything* rather than voluntarily spend time around him…

Beck got up and moved through the kitchen. Since she'd left, staying still had become a real issue. Which was funny because he always joked that he never liked to be still. He was always planning things. Going on adventures. Seeking new things.

Running from his parents' life—if Vi was to be believed.

"She isn't right. I'm not running."

Toaster tilted her head and let out a bark. She was sweet company but not the best conversationalist.

Looking at the closed door to his parents' study, he crossed his arms. He could march in there right now, look at that bucket of old photos and prove her wrong.

"I don't need to."

Again, Toaster tilted her head.

"Sorry, girl. Just talking to myself." Beck started toward the door. He'd look at the one picture. The boring pic. It was all he ever needed to remind himself that he wasn't going to follow their path.

Stepping into the room, he took a deep breath and looked at the picture. His dad was looking at his mom. It was the exact same as it had been for as long as he could remember.

Her in a bright dress, the sun hitting just right on her face. His father looking at her. The rest of the world gone. Nothing about it had changed.

But…

Beck ran his hand over the glass. His father's face was brilliant. He raced toward the picture he kept of his father in the living room. Him on top of a mountain.

Beck had climbed that mountain right after college graduation. Stood on the top and had another hiker snap his picture re-creating his father's photo. He kept meaning to hang it next to his dad's.

Now, looking at the two pictures of his father, it was easy to see which one radiated happiness. And it wasn't the one of him alone on a summit.

No.

He moved to the hallway photos, each was the same, his dad looked fine, happy even. But not content.

Reaching for his phone, he pulled up the photo Callie sent him after the first time he brought Vi to the gym. She'd told him congrats—and that she was retiring from trying to find him a date.

He stared at the picture.

People had always told him how much he looked like his mother. He had his father's height, but his facial features and hair were all his mother. But in this image, looking at Violet like there was no one else in his world, he was his father's spitting image.

He loved her. And rather than telling Violet that he couldn't see a life without her in it—instead of inviting her on the adventures he wanted to take—he'd let her walk away.

How did one make up for that?

How did he even begin to show her how sorry he was?

The idea formed quickly. He wasn't sure it was possible but for Vi—for Vi he'd do anything.

The image of them standing on the agility course, love pouring from him long before he'd even realized it, bolstered him as he started trying to track down the one person who might be willing to help him.

Soft music poured through the speakers in Nancy's car. Violet had expected to spend the entire trip to Boston answering agility questions. Instead, Nancy had asked how she was doing then asked if Violet minded classical music.

The music choice wasn't her favorite, but Nancy was kind enough to offer her a ride. And she hadn't peppered her with any questions about Beck.

Violet bit her lip as his name echoed in her mind. Five days into forever without him. And it hurt more than she could have ever imagined.

And she'd been left at the altar.

Following the demise of her engagement, she'd been hurt. Embarrassed. Mad at herself for not recognizing the signs that Thomas was all wrong for her.

But the soul crushing emptiness she felt now hadn't appeared.

"Did I ever tell you why I got into agility?" Nancy's question offered a nice respite.

"No." Violet was sure Nancy knew she'd never told her. She was trying to distract her.

The gym owner might be more than a little too uptight about the gym, and her rules for trainers were actively keeping them away—though she'd loosened them after Vi had pointed out some of the issue. But she'd offered the ride to Boston quietly without pressure.

"What made you get into the sport?" Vi smiled and turned her attention to Nancy.

"My ex-husband." Nancy laughed. A true belly laugh that made the crow's-feet around the older woman's eyes deepen.

"Your ex-husband was into the sport?" Violet had seen all sorts of things when she worked in Miami. One couple had even gone to court over who maintained custody of the dog.

"No. He hated dogs."

"Good riddance then." Violet chuckled. Thomas was an ass, but the man genuinely liked animals. It was his only redeeming quality.

"Exactly." Nancy nodded. "I got a border collie the second we separated. He told me he'd file for divorce if I didn't get rid of the dog."

"Men." Vi rolled her eyes.

"I told him that was not the threat he thought it was." Nancy quickly looked back at Oliver.

"Good for you."

"Yes. Lilly was my baby, but as a first-time dog owner border collies are…" Nancy put her finger on her chin.

"A lot." Violet finished the thought. "There is a reason I never recommend that breed to new pet parents. They are bred to work."

"Yes. Lilly was a lot. I started driving to an agility gym two hours away." Nancy started tapping her fingers on the steering wheel. "It was fun to learn. Lilly and I had the best time."

"It's a great sport for humans and dogs."

"I fell in love with a trainer." Nancy let out a sigh. "You remind me of him sometimes. So professional. So knowledgeable but focused on the dogs and people not the trophies. But in other ways you are me. I can see it so easily. Maybe it's a benefit of age or something."

Vi didn't know what to say.

"We had a wild affair. The best six months of my life." Nancy blew out a breath.

Now she wished she'd said something. She looked at her lap, not sure how to end this conversation. The feelings she was not burying well on her own were now ready to spill over in the car with Nancy.

"He was my great love and I let him go. I was so worried that I might lose the independence I gained from my ex. I put all my fears from the relationship on him—something he didn't deserve. When I realized I loved him, I pulled away instead of running toward him."

"Nancy—"

"I opened the gym four years after the last time I saw him. He passed less than two weeks after our final fight, a car accident."

"I'm so sorry."

Nancy didn't look at her as she kept spilling her heartbreak. "I'd give up anything for those two weeks. Anything for more time. My ex got to win in the end because I was too stubborn to start over."

The older woman took a deep breath. "I don't know what happened with you and Beck. And it is the definition of not my business. But you are not the same person you were before him. I don't know why and I don't need to. And maybe he did something unforgivable."

"He didn't."

Nancy bit her lip, like she was weighing saying something else.

"The past is there to learn from, but those who hurt us can jade things they have no business jading." Nancy looked at the radio and shook her head. "No more classical. Time for some hard rock."

The heavy beats blasted through the car, and there was no way to have a conversation. Mentally she sent a simple thank you to Nancy.

Violet had packed up her things—shocked at the number of items she'd actually moved into Beck's place. She would not have said they were living together, but her car's trunk was full of stuff that she'd transitioned to his space without even thinking.

And then there was the stained glass. She packed that first. Not that Beck knew it.

Everything else at his place was technically replaceable. But not that key chain. She'd grabbed that first in case he woke while she was busy.

Because I didn't trust him.

She'd let her fear take control. A fear she'd developed from Thomas and thrown over Beck.

They'd needed to have a conversation. She'd needed to ask if he saw a future with her. Needed to work through his issues fearing marriage. All of that was needed.

But she'd packed up first. Guaranteed the outcome of the conversation. For someone who craved loyalty and steadiness, she'd walked first.

"How close are we to the facility?" Violet called over the rock music.

"Just under an hour. Plenty of time to work up a speech." She winked at her, then started singing along to the ballad blasting from her radio.

It's here. Standing by concessions will leave in five if you are not here.

Beck read Dove's text and took off at a sprint. Luckily Toaster was so well trained she kept up with him perfectly.

The concessions came into sight and Dove was standing there looking nervously around, holding a package wrapped in brown paper.

He held out a hand. "Is that the tablecloth? I can't tell you how much I appreciate this, Dove. I know this must be awkward for you."

She passed it over and nodded. "I didn't realize that it

was— Look, just tell her to keep it off social media, okay? He won't notice it's gone if no one draws attention to it. I don't know why he even took it to be honest. It's not really his style of decor."

Beck was pretty sure he knew why, but he wasn't going to say so in front of Dove after she'd done him this favor.

"Thanks again. It will mean a lot to Vi."

"Sure. You don't need to tell her how you got it though. Just keep my name out of it, okay? I don't need any problems."

"Of course."

As she spotted her doppelgänger weaving through the crowds looking for Beck, Dove looked startled and quickly melted away into the background before he could say any more. Delighted to see her, Beck made his way toward Violet and the world disappeared as she wrapped her arms around him.

"I'm sorry, Beck." She whispered the words in his ear and he was stunned.

"You have nothing to apologize for. You were right. I was so terrified of becoming a homebody, but I looked at the picture of my parents again. You were right. They were alive when they were together. Truly alive. They didn't need more."

"But you do. And that's okay." Violet wrapped her hand through his.

"I want more adventures, but I want you beside me while I take them. While we take them. I love you, Violet. I love you so much. I should have told you so many times. But mostly I should have told you when you were so worried about my reaction to people talking marriage. That issue is mine not yours, and I put it on you." Beck ran his hand down her back, so grateful to just have her here.

"I love you too. And you weren't the only one letting your

personal stuff get in the way. I was looking for any sign I might get left. That you might not want what I wanted. I let fear rule me and I took the first chance to leave so didn't get hurt. That wasn't fair." Violet's hand cupped his cheek. "I love you."

"I love you too, Vi. And I've got something for you. Something you've been missing for a long time." Her eyes fell on the package in his hands and she opened her mouth, then shook her head. "No. Is that…?"

He passed her the package and watched her remove the brown wrapping. "I will admit that I got this because I was hoping to use it to win you back."

Vi laughed. "You don't have to win me back, but—" Her fingers gently touched the cloth and tears sprang to her eyes. "How did you…?"

"Oh, don't you worry about that. I have my ways."

"Oh thank you, Beck. Thank you so much."

Beck's lips brushed hers, and Toaster let out a bark. "If I wouldn't be letting the team down, I would say we could get out of here." He pulled her even closer.

"I say we go beat Thomas's team, then spend the night making it up to each other. Maybe stay an extra night in Boston. The Holiday Market at Snowport is already open, and I hear it is quite the place to be this time of year."

"That sounds like the perfect plan." Beck kissed her cheek. "The perfect plan indeed."

EPILOGUE

"WHAT DO YOU THINK?" Vi held up the secret project she'd been working on at Mitch's studio. The one that Beck was not allowed to peek at. The one that she wasn't 100 percent sure he'd like.

Beck put his hand over his mouth. To hide his horror?

"Vi." Tears clouded his eyes as he stared at the stained-glass window. A re-creation of his parents' favorite photo.

The "boring one," as Beck still referred to it. Though now he said it with a grin on his face.

"If you don't like it—"

"I love it."

"Oh good. Because if you hated it after it took me nearly a year to work out, I might have burst into tears right here." Vi chuckled as Beck stepped toward her.

They'd lived in his home for almost three years now. And she was certain he'd love this gift on the day she'd started it. But as the image took shape and she was framing it, part of her had feared the argument they'd had years ago regarding the photo might resurface.

A wild fear. Totally baseless.

"I do wish Mom and Dad had gotten to see it." He took the framed glass from her hands and put it up on the mantel next to the image of him and Vi skydiving last year on vacation in Florida.

"We are going to have to put it in an actual window. Don't suppose you know a class that will teach us how to install a full-size stained-glass window?" Beck reached for her, pulling her close.

"No, but I bet Mitch can help us figure it out." Violet leaned her head against his shoulder. The man who'd taught them stained-glass techniques was a jack-of-all-trades, and his home had many stained-glass windows in the panes.

"You really think they'd have liked it?" She'd never get to meet the lovely people that raised the man she loved more than anything. She hoped they liked the woman he'd chosen as a life partner.

"They'd have loved it." Beck kissed the top of her head. "Which brings me to another thing they'd have loved."

He turned and got down on one knee.

Vi pulled her hands over her mouth as tears filled her eyes. "Yes. Yes. A million times yes!"

"I haven't asked anything yet, Vi." Beck had tears in his eyes too as he looked up at her.

She pursed her lips, even though he couldn't see them behind her hands to keep her mouth shut long enough for him to ask the question.

"Will you marry me, Vi?"

Before she could say anything, Toaster and Bear bounded into the room, saw Beck on the floor and took full advantage. The dogs knocked him over, and he let out a grunt as the two covered him with kisses.

Vi couldn't have stopped the belly laughs if she wanted to. Tears were pouring down her face; happiness filled the whole scene.

She'd meant what she'd told him years ago. She didn't need

a ring or a certificate. Marriage and a life partner were one and the same to her as long as they had each other.

This was the life she'd craved. A happy home with a partner who adored her.

"Can you stop laughing long enough to answer?" Beck called from the literal dog pile.

"Yes." She giggled a little more, then said, "Heel." Toaster was immediately at her side. Bear looked at her, nuzzled Beck one more time, then sashayed over to her side.

Beck stood and she held out her hand. "I love you, Vi. I love you so much. In the exciting times. The boring times. And every single moment in between."

* * * * *

If you enjoyed this story, check out these other great reads from Juliette Hyland

One-Night Baby with Her Best Friend
Dating His Irresistible Rival
Her Secret Baby Confession
A Puppy on the 34th Ward

All available now!

COMING SOON!

We really hope you enjoyed reading this book.
If you're looking for more romance
be sure to head to the shops when
new books are available on

Thursday 21st November

To see which titles are coming soon, please visit
millsandboon.co.uk/nextmonth

MILLS & BOON

MILLS & BOON®

Coming next month

MELTING DR GRUMPY'S FROZEN HEART
Scarlet Wilson

This guy didn't know her background. He didn't know why she was here.

For Skye, cancer research was personal. But she didn't know his background, or what had made him do years of training and decide that oncology was the place he wanted to work. She wasn't here to make an enemy. But from the expression on his face, she was doubting she was making a friend.

She decided to push in another direction. 'You know,' she said breezily, 'I am a huge Christmas fan. You'll learn that over the next few weeks. My favourite movie is The Grinch. I'd hate for people to start calling you that.'

The edges of his mouth hinted upwards and he gave a sigh, as his eyebrows raised. The expression had the hint of a cheeky teenager about it. 'My nickname is Dr Grumpy, and yes, I know that,' he replied in that delicious thick Irish accent.

'And mine is Miss Sunshine,' she replied, holding her hand out to his.

Jay Bannerman didn't even hide the groan that came out his mouth as he shook her hand. 'This is going to be a disaster, isn't it?'

For a second – at least in Skye's head – things froze. She was captured by the man sitting in front of her. Now she'd stopped focusing on everything else she realised just how handsome he was. Discounting the fact that every time he spoke that lilting accent sent a whole host of vibrations down her spine, even if he hadn't opened his mouth, and she'd seen him in a bar, this guy was hot.

Skye didn't mix business with pleasure. She'd never been interested in dating her colleagues.

But at least he was semi-smiling now, and she would take that.

Continue reading

MELTING DR GRUMPY'S FROZEN HEART
Scarlet Wilson

Available next month
millsandboon.co.uk

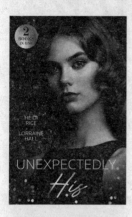
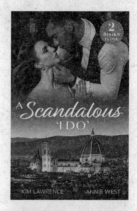
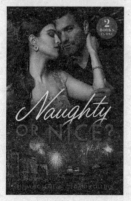
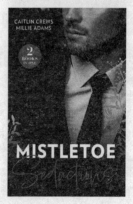

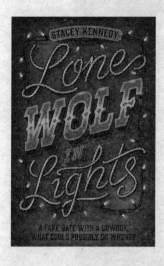 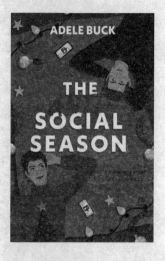

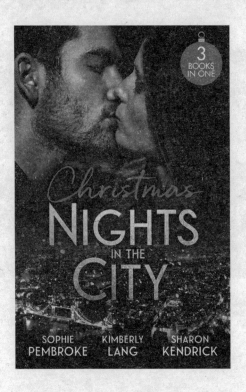

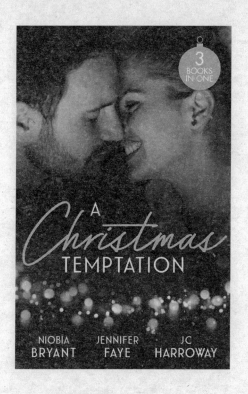

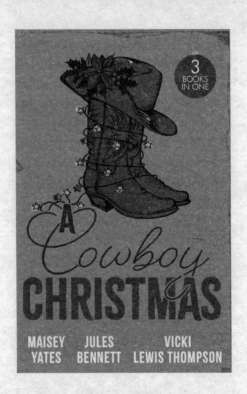

MILLS & BOON

THE HEART OF ROMANCE

A ROMANCE FOR EVERY READER

MODERN
Prepare to be swept off your feet by sophisticated, sexy and seductive heroes, in some of the world's most glamourous and romantic locations, where power and passion collide.

HISTORICAL
Escape with historical heroes from time gone by. Whether your passion is for wicked Regency Rakes, muscled Vikings or rugged Highlanders, awaken the romance of the past.

MEDICAL
Set your pulse racing with dedicated, delectable doctors in the high-pressure world of medicine, where emotions run high and passion, comfort and love are the best medicine.

True Love
Celebrate true love with tender stories of heartfelt romance, from the rush of falling in love to the joy a new baby can bring, and a focus on the emotional heart of a relationship.

HEROES
The excitement of a gripping thriller, with intense romance at its heart. Resourceful, true-to-life women and strong, fearless men face danger and desire - a killer combination!

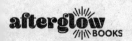
From showing up to glowing up, these characters are on the path to leading their best lives and finding romance along the way – with plenty of sizzling spice!

To see which titles are coming soon, please visit

millsandboon.co.uk/nextmonth

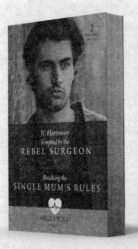
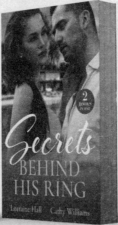
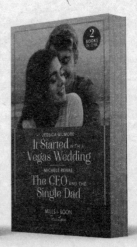